What is Importance of Healthy Nutrition Pyramids?

Healthy Nutrition Facts and Tips

with Counting Calories Guide

Andrew Roman

Table of Contents

Introduction

More and more people are looking for a healthy way of life. After all, we all want to live a long time and enjoy ourselves as much as we can. Healthy nutrition is part of this journey. This is where *OMG! What is Healthy Nutrition?* comes to the rescue.

The purpose of this book is to teach you about nutrition and living healthy. There's a lot of information out there about this topic and a lot of it isn't true or it's badly perceived. So, use this guide to navigate through all of this misinformation and learn from genuine sources that come from science, research, and experience.

With the help of this book you will gain an understanding about the fundamental concepts of healthy nutrition. You will learn about the food guide pyramids. (Yes, there are more than one!) You will find out the truth behind many of the most popular myths and misconceptions about diet, weight loss, and nutrition. And most importantly, you will learn how to eat right and have fun at the same time. So let's go on this journey of discovery together and begin a new healthy life!

Why Should You Trust this Book

Hi! My name's Andrew and I welcome you to my book about healthy living. You are probably asking yourself right now "why should I believe what this guy has to say when there are countless other resources?" Skepticism is good to have, especially nowadays with so many food myths floating around the Internet.

Not that long ago I asked myself that very same question when learning about healthy nutrition. I'm a health-obsessed author from New York nowadays, but before that, I used to focus on climbing the management ladder in a number of big shot corporations. As you can probably imagine, that ruined my health. I gained a great deal of weight, and my quality of life dropped the more I climbed the ladder. Ambition is a hell of a drug, but stress and being overworked was killing me. So, what changed?

I began to study nutrition and the reasons why I was gaining so much weight. Learning all the facts that I used to ignore has opened my eyes. I started making changes immediately and I lost 40 pounds without gaining it all back. That's when I realized that there are many people who are in the same boat I was. So, I continued studying the subject and started helping people through the power of the written word.

I want to share my experience with you and point you to real scientific sources that don't try to sell you the next magic weight loss pill. I'm not making you any false promises. At the end of the day, losing weight and eating healthy is all up to you. All I can do is enlighten you and give you all the tools you need to make the right decisions. So, sit down a while, and learn how healthy nutrition is the key to a good life.

Chapter 1: Manage Your Health with Healthy Nutrition

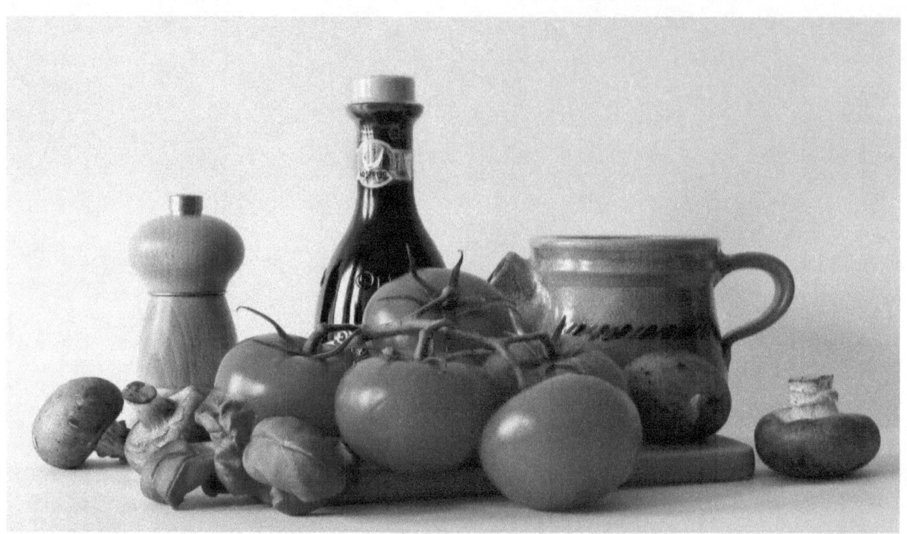

In the past couple of decades nutritionists and researchers have made it clear that a healthy diet is key to a good living standard and a long life. It's difficult to go through an entire day without reading a story, an article, or listening to someone talking about health, nutrition, and weight loss. If you log into Facebook or any other social media you consume right now, you will probably see such a post. The news that we can improve our lives, limit the chances of getting cancer, lose weight, get ripped, and look younger through a healthy diet is now familiar to all of us. Due to decades of research mand study, we now have the knowledge to improve our nutrition without sacrificing the food we love so much.

However, despite the visual bombardment we experience on nutrition and weight loss, people continue to eat what they shouldn't. Obesity is becoming a bigger problem than before, especially now with teenagers and young adults. So why do people still cling to an unhealthy lifestyle? In most cases the guidelines to a healthy diet are complex. What the government and the universities publish is just too complex for the average reader. Most of us naturally question what we are told, so we tend to ask questions like "why" when it comes to changing the food we love so much. In addition, food is equal to pleasure, and few people are willing to give up on fools that comfort and relieve stress.

With that being said, in this chapter we are going to discuss how healthy nutrition can help you with your health and weight loss. You will learn the "why" and by the end you will realize that managing your health through nutrition isn't such a daunting task after all.

Optimization Is Key

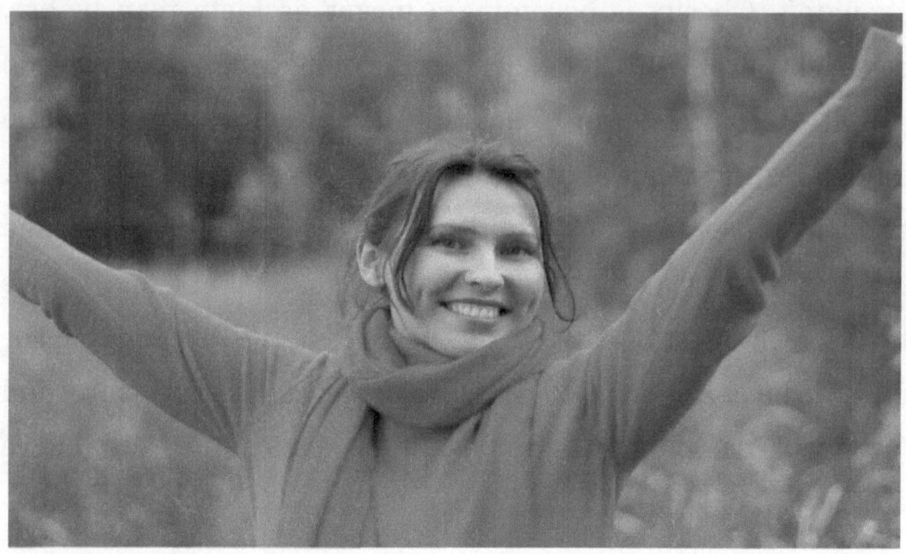

Have you walked past a cake shop recently, looked through the window, and suddenly decided to treat yourself with a lovely slice of cheesecake or a muffin? Have you walked in front of a bakery and the smell of freshly baked croissants lured you in? On a daily basis we are surrounded by so many choices and options. There is so much food to pick from and it's all around us. All that it takes is a choice.

We make choices every single day. These decisions depend on our culture, lifestyle, knowledge, goals, moods, and so much more. And every choice has a consequence. Our ancient ancestors didn't have this luxury. All they had to choose from was food that they could find themselves, that they could hunt or gather. Nowadays, with all of our technological advances and the global migration, we can find pretty much every type of food from any corner of the world. We don't depend on what we gather. Instead, we get to enjoy our favorite Indian dishes in Canada or an Apple Strudel in South Africa.

There are no limits to food, so making the right choice has become infinitely more difficult. It's not easy to choose the food that improves our health or offers us the right nutrients we're missing. This is a problem and we need to overcome it.

Every person in the world needs the same nutrients. Nutrients are fuel for our bodies, for our very lives, they sustain us and it's up to us to fill the tank the right way. After all, you don't want to put diesel in a car that runs on gasoline or the engine's going to die in no time and need some serious "detox" in order to function again. The amounts of each nutrient is what makes us unique because it all depends on our age, sex, current physique, goals, and so on. For instance, pregnant women and bodybuilders need foods that are much richer in nutrients. This is where nutrition optimization comes in.

A general guide for the intake of nutrients was developed by various nutritional scientists. This guide is known as the Dietary Reference Intakes, and it's important because it specifies the optimal nutritional guidelines based on your sex and age. If you do a quick search you will find that there are detailed DRI for each age group and then further divided for each sex. But how did scientists figure out these optimal nutrition requirements?

This story starts during the Second World War, when nutrition experts were tasked to figure out the dietary necessities of the soldiers so that they could be in an optimal condition. Since then, the guidelines that started with the military kept being updated by new generations of scientists with the help of new technologies and medical progress.

Nowadays, the research about nutrition is focused on preventing a wide variety of diseases, as well as reducing the risk of developing certain illnesses such as various forms of heart diseases and cancer. This is how, in 1997, the Recommended Dietary Allowance came to be. This guideline tells us what we need to eat in order to prevent a wide range of health problems. It's very detailed and we are not going to dive into it. Otherwise, you might feel overwhelmed and move on. What you need to take from it, however, is the fact that four of the 10 main causes of death in the US are strongly affected, and related to your diet (IHME, 2019). By optimizing your nutrition intake and living healthier overall, you can significantly reduce your chances of suffering from heart diseases, cancer, stroke, and diabetes.

Eating Often and Dietary Education

You already understand the importance of nutrition and why you need to learn how to optimize it. However, the second question is how often should you eat? Many people don't even ask themselves this question because they eat when they're hungry.

Chances are, you do the same, because after all the body screams it's hungry when it's looking for more nutrients, right? Well, that is partially true. For instance, think of the time you suddenly get a craving for red meat or spinach. That is often a sign that you lack iron and your body is looking for foods that are rich in that particular nutrient. However, your body is also influenced by your desire to experience pleasure, happiness, and relaxation. Food does that to you. It relieves your anxiety, it gives you a moment of joy, and it generally relaxes you.

Because of the problems mentioned above, we need guidelines. We need information so that we can make the right choice and not just blindly follow our cravings. Our brains get pleasure from fats and sugars because of an ancient instinct to fatten up for our survival, among other things, however, we cannot allow ourselves to follow this instinct anymore. This is one of the reasons why a number of research institutions came up with the five times a day meal plan. The new plan was actually designed to teach people about eating vegetables and fruit more often. In some cases, it was advised to have up to nine meals a day, mostly consisting of fruits and veggies. But, let's face it, who has the time to each, much less prepare or cook five to nine small meals on a daily basis?

Eating often, especially fruit and vegetables, have improved the overall health statistics. The education efforts of governments have led people to consume a lot less saturated fat, and eat more fruit and vegetables. This alone has shown that eating healthy isn't just about the amount of calories you consume. It's important to get the right type of nutrients. It's not the same for your heart and blood vessels if you eat an apple, or its equivalent in potato chips that are soaked in saturated fats.

Brief Guide to a Healthy Diet

Eating the right things is important, but this isn't THE solution to all of our health problems caused by our eating habits. In order to live healthy, we need to use different tools. To stick with our car analogy from earlier, it's not enough to keep feeling the car with gas, we also need to take care of it by changing its oil, and making sure everything is according to specs. Our bodies work the same way. So, one of the first things we need to sort out is maintaining a healthy weight through fitness.

We all know by now that being overweight isn't healthy. No matter what leads a person to be obese, that isn't good for the heart, and he or she can develop diabetes and other health issues. And if you are overweight, you should combine a healthy eating plan with plenty of physical activity. This can be a problem to many nowadays. Just think of all the office jobs out there. You might be working in an office yourself. What does your day look like? If you get out of bed, shower, eat, drive to work, spend 9 hours at a desk, drive back home, watch Netflix, sleep, and repeat, then chances are your body isn't fit. Just keep in mind that you can also be skinny, or at a normal body weight, but that doesn't mean you're healthy. Too many people think they're fine just because they aren't overweight.

Exercising is crucial. Fitness is to nutrition what Yin is to Yang. We need physical activity to keep the heart healthy, to maintain muscle mass, and to get a dose of energy. Not exercising can make us feel constantly tired and lethargic. However, we can easily fix this!

If you see yourself in the image we just discussed, all you need to do is add a 30 min period of physical activity per day. If you are particularly sedentary, then you can start with even less activity and gradually increase it. This isn't as scary as it sounds though. You don't necessarily have to pick up jogging at 6 in the morning, and you don't need to pay for a gym membership either. All you need to do is make small changes throughout your day. For instance, you can walk to the office if you don't live more than half an hour away. You can also ditch the car for a bicycle. You'd be surprised how much distance you can cover on a bike, and it's quite a bit less expensive. Burn calories and fat instead of gas. It's good for you, and nature as well, which is an added bonus.

If walking or cycling is out of the question, you can do numerous exercises at home, or even at the office, with nothing but your own bodyweight. Check out some videos on home fitness on Youtube.

Once you have your fitness routine in check, you need to take a look at your choice in food. Here you can use the food pyramid as a guide (we will discuss this much more in the next chapter), and choose a wide variety of nutritious foods.

Did you know that your body needs at least around 40 nutrients in order to function at optimal level? Sounds like a lot, but if you keep your diet varied, you can gain all of them. In addition, a varied diet will also keep you from getting bored. Normally we associate diets and the word "healthy" with boring. But that's just because of bad advertising and your parents yelling at you to eat all your food, even if you didn't like it (my nemesis was broccoli). It doesn't have to be that way, not today with so many ways of cooking every possible ingredient. Just think of how many cultures there are on Earth and each one has developed a different way of cooking things like broccoli. Exciting!

To quickly gain control over your diet, you should start by selecting a wide variety of whole grains. Grains are rich in fiber, minerals, vitamins, and various other organic compounds that are crucial for minimizing the risk of heart disease and other problems that appear with age. Next, you need fruits and vegetables. They are rich in nutrients and don't have any fat. Just make sure you eat them instead of drinking them. That orange juice might be tasty, but you're leaving behind most nutrients that are actually found in the pulp and inner linings of the fruit. When you drink a few oranges for instance, instead of eating one, you might still get some nutrients, but you are actually consuming mostly sugars and empty calories. So, eat your fruits and veggies, or "drink" them whole, not just squeezed.

Finally, you need to make the right choices as with anything in life. You need to start paying close attention to the nutritional content label on the pack of whatever you buy. If you need to learn the nutritional value of various fruits, since they don't come with a label usually, you are a Google search away from the answer. Simply type something like "nutritional value of an orange." Other than that, you can stick to things you probably already know, like fats, sugars, salt, and alcohol being usually bad for you if not consumed sparingly.

Summary

In this chapter we glanced at what eating healthy means and why we need to pay attention to nutrition in general. Before you start making significant changes to your life and to your diet, you need to take a step back and analyze where you are right now. Be honest with yourself and identify the problems so you can address them one at a time. Just keep in mind that nutrition is an aspect of your entire lifestyle. When you work on making healthy changes to get the proper nutrition your body and brain need, you are making a long-term commitment. So, take your time to form a relationship with yourself and the food you eat.

Chapter 2: The Food Pyramid

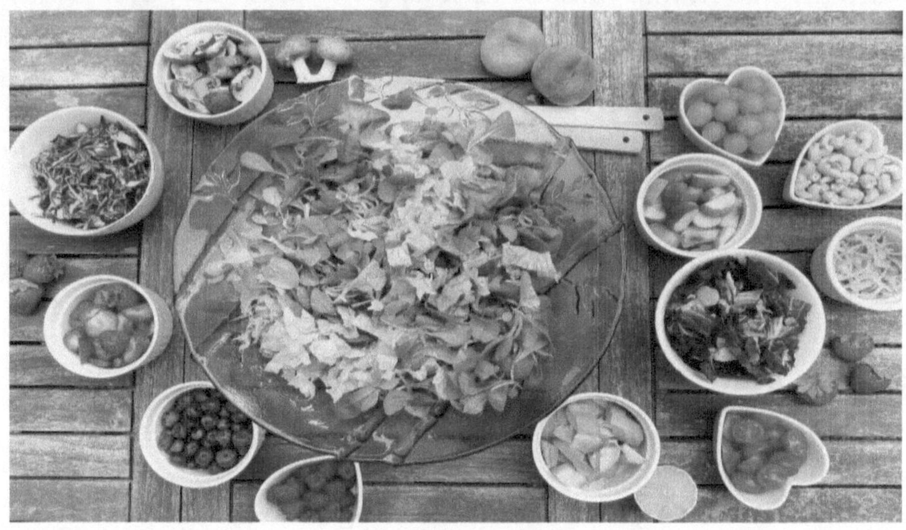

Learning about all the nutrients you need can be quite tedious. Just imagine memorizing the 40+ things your body requires, the food items that contain them, and then checking each ingredient at the store to see the percentage of what you get. Doesn't sound fun, does it? Good thing we can skip all that. It's still good to know the basics and what's most important, however, to help you get started quicker, you can use the food guide pyramid.

The food pyramid, or food guide pyramid, or nutrition pyramid (it comes under many names), was designed to help the consumer get a better idea of what he or she needs to eat to stay in shape. The pyramid is very easy to understand. You have sugars, fats and oils at the top, meaning you should not eat much of them. Then you have dairy products like cottage cheese and yogurt, as well as protein-rich foods like meats, beans, lentils, and tofu, followed by fruits and vegetables. At the base of the pyramid we have the grains, whether we're talking about rice, cereals, or whole-wheat bread. The higher a product is in the pyramid, the less you should consume it. However, that doesn't mean you should ignore it. For example, eliminating all fat from your diet is bad for your body. So, don't go from one extreme to another, even if you're trying to lose weight. Everything needs to be consumed in moderation and combined with physical activity. Remember that and you are well on your way to living healthy.

Servings and Variety

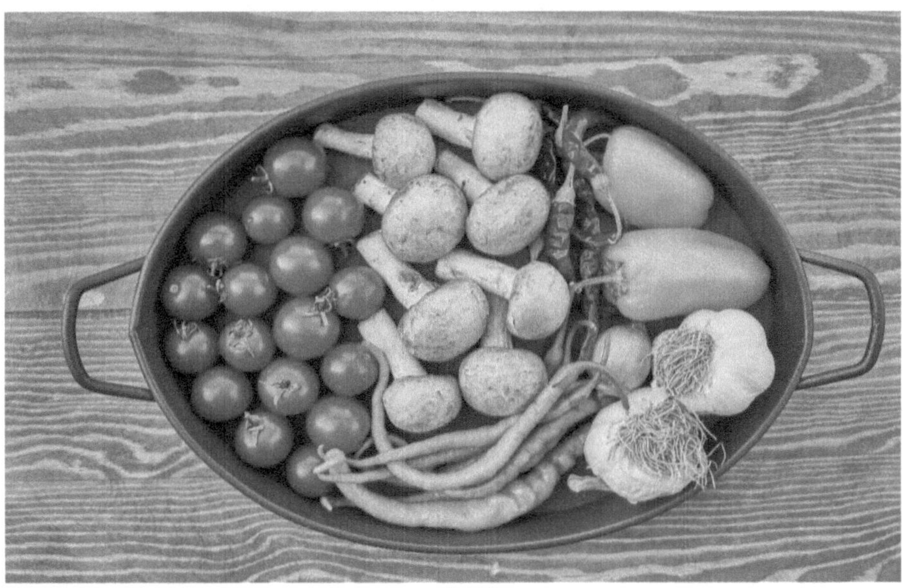

The food guide pyramid is useful, but it won't help you much if you don't know how to divide the servings. As mentioned, you need to break down your diet into the major food groups: grains, fruits, vegetables, dairy products, meats and protein-rich foods, and fats, oils and sugars. Then you need to plan the number of servings for each category. Sounds a bit like there's too much math, right? Unfortunately, you need to go through the planning stage, but the good news is that you only need to do so once.

The number of servings is calculated based on age, sex, and physical activity. For instance, an active woman can easily consume around 2,200 calories in total per day without gaining weight. However, if you have a more sedentary life, and you spend most of your time at a desk, you might have to plan to eat only around 1,600 calories per day. These numbers aren't set in stone though. There are just too many things that affect how many calories you burn. We all know that skinny guy or girl who seems to be eating constantly but not gaining any weight. Others are less fortunate and have a slower metabolism. That is why you'll need to experiment a bit, however, you can use the guidelines as a general idea, not as a rule.

Here's an example of a typical, modern female adult's diet that consists of 1,600 calories:

1. Grains: Six servings distributed throughout the day
2. Fruits: Two servings, usually as in-between snacks or dessert
3. Vegetables: Three servings

4. Dairy: Two servings, unless you are a young adult up to 24 years old, or pregnant (hen you should add three servings)

5. Meats / Protein: Two servings

If you find yourself in a more active category, you need to increase the number of servings. However, there are some exceptions when it comes to healthy nutrition. For instance, if you follow a 2,200 calorie diet, then you will significantly boost the quantity of grains, fruits and vegetables you eat, but the dairy and meat servings stay the same. This is due to the high fat content in the last two groups. The general idea is to consume some fat because it's very important for your health, but fatty foods should not represent more than a third of your calorie requirements. So, if you think you should eat more because you're active, try to stick to a higher variety of fruits and vegetables instead of having an extra burger. Your body will be grateful, especially as you grow older. Now let's get back to the pyramid.

Pyramids and Diets

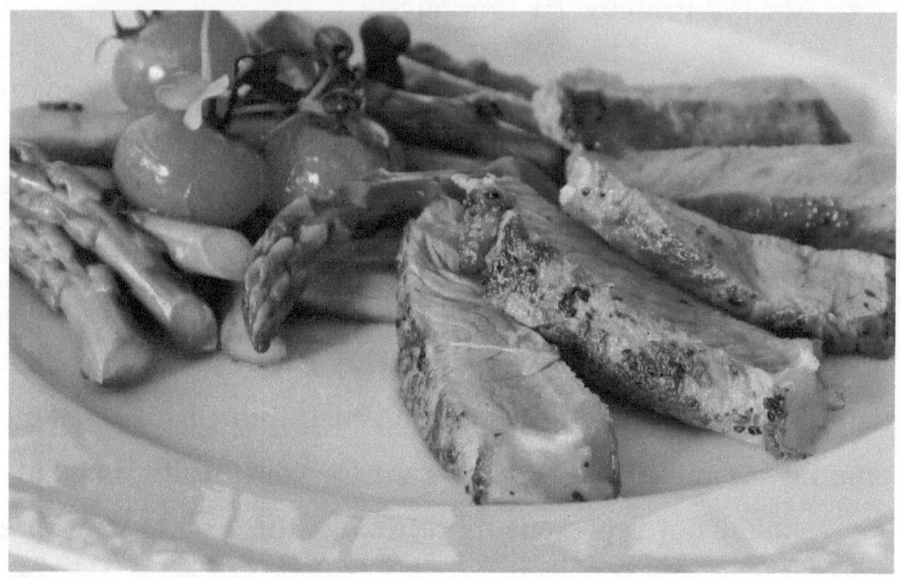

So far, we only talked about the nutritional guide pyramid that nearly everyone is familiar with these days. While that pyramid can serve you well in your quest for a healthy lifestyle, there are other pyramids as well. New food guide pyramids were developed over time to suit each kind of diet. Why? Simply because someone living in Asia, or in the Mediterranean region, doesn't have access to the same types of food.

Each one of these pyramids can be useful to you no matter where you're from. You can even use the information to combine the food types in order to create an even more varied, but still balanced, diet. In this section we are going to briefly explore a few other food guide pyramids, such as the Mediterranean and Vegan Pyramids, to add some more variation to your lifestyle.

The Mediterranean Diet Pyramid

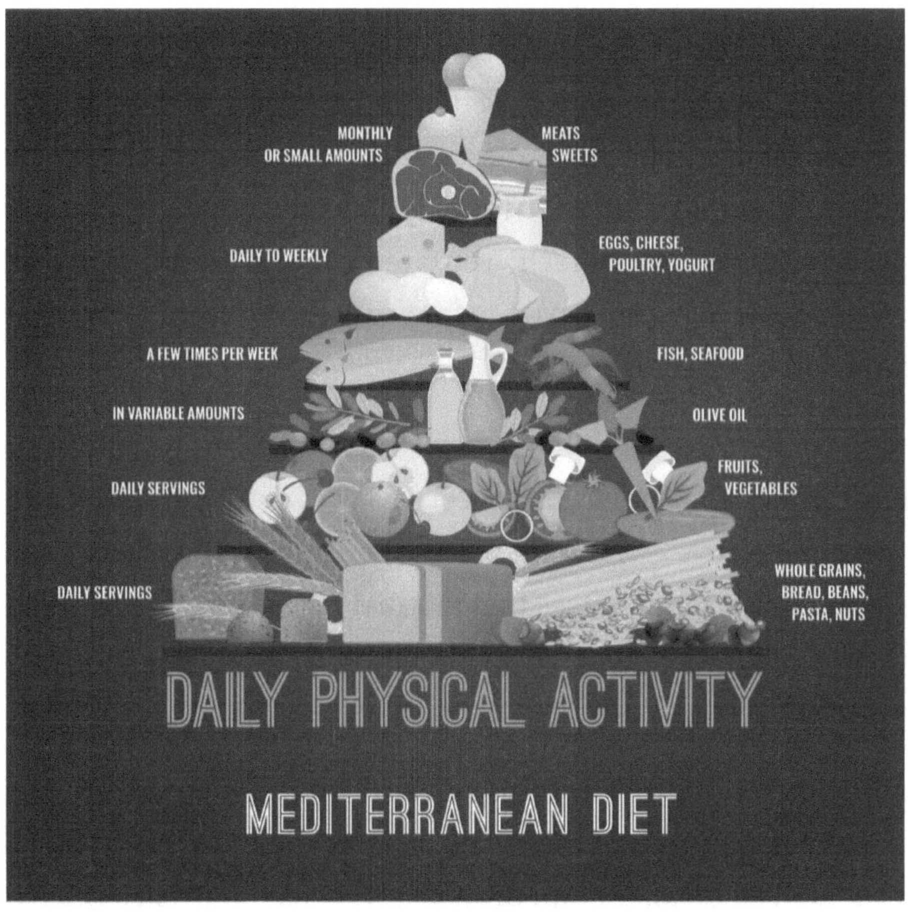

You probably already heard about the Mediterranean diet. It's been making quite a buzz among nutritionists and doctors alike, because statistically, those who follow it seem to live longer. There are scientific studies that show that people living in the Mediterranean region have a prolonged life span, in general. Check out this article in the Journal of Nutrition, published by Cambridge University Press, if you're interested in the details.

We won't get too technical in this book (British Journal of Nutrition, 2018).

This pyramid and diet is interesting because at its base it starts with the recommendation of being physically active. It also advises people to be social during meals and to share them with others. Naturally, while you should indeed workout, if you like peaceful meals by yourself, you aren't forced to interact with other people. It's ok to have a more private relationship with your food and to relax on your own.

Next comes the bulk of the pyramid. This segment will make up most of your diet and it consists of a wide variety of grains, fruits, vegetables, olive oil, legumes, seeds, nuts, as well as herbs and spices. You can already see that this diet focuses on a much wider variety than the general food pyramid. Even healthy oils, especially olive oil, is part of the base of the pyramid, not the top.

Moving upward, we have fish and seafood. In the previous diet, this category is part of the meats or protein part of the pyramid. That food guide focuses on protein as the main nutrient which is found in these products, as well as in lentils and beans. However, fish is a very different protein source when compared to meat. It's usually lower in calories, unless you use ingredients like oil and flour to cook it, and it contains other healthy nutrients that meat doesn't, such as Omega-3 fats. (The exception to this rule is grass-fed beef, which is rich in Omega-3 fats.) These fats are essential and unlike other types of fats, they are healthy. However, since variety is the car that drives you towards the healthy nutrition bank, you should make sure to consume fish and seafood around twice a week.

Next up, we have the dairy products, together with poultry and eggs. Another important difference. Cheese, yogurt, and poultry products should be eaten often, but in small portions distributed throughout the day. For instance, you can have a serving of yogurt as a snack in between meals.

Red meat is rarely eaten in the Mediterranean diet. That is why it's found at the top of the pyramid together with sweets. So, if you follow this diet, and you're crazy about juicy steaks or ground beef, you'll have to adjust accordingly. Remember that grass-fed beef is much healthier than corn-fed beef, due to the difference in healthy Omega-3 fats.

Next to all the food, the pyramid advises drinking a lot of water. This aspect is often ignored, and many people suffer due to not staying hydrated. Getting bloated? Are your ankles sometimes swollen? Chances are you don't drink enough water. Why is that? Even if you don't feel thirsty, your body needs water for many of its internal processes like digesting food or regulating body temperature. When you don't drink enough, your body retains that water. So, if you think you have this problem, you should drink more, not less. Some people falsely believe that they will gain water weight if they hydrate too often. What actually happens is the opposite.

Finally, there's some good news if you are a wine lover. This pyramid recommends wine, especially red wine, to be drunk regularly, but in moderation. After all, you know how much Italians love wine. That might be the secret to why they live longer than others. So, if you like wine, why risk it? Have a nice glass of red with your dinner and savor what life has to offer.

The Healthy Vegan Food Pyramid

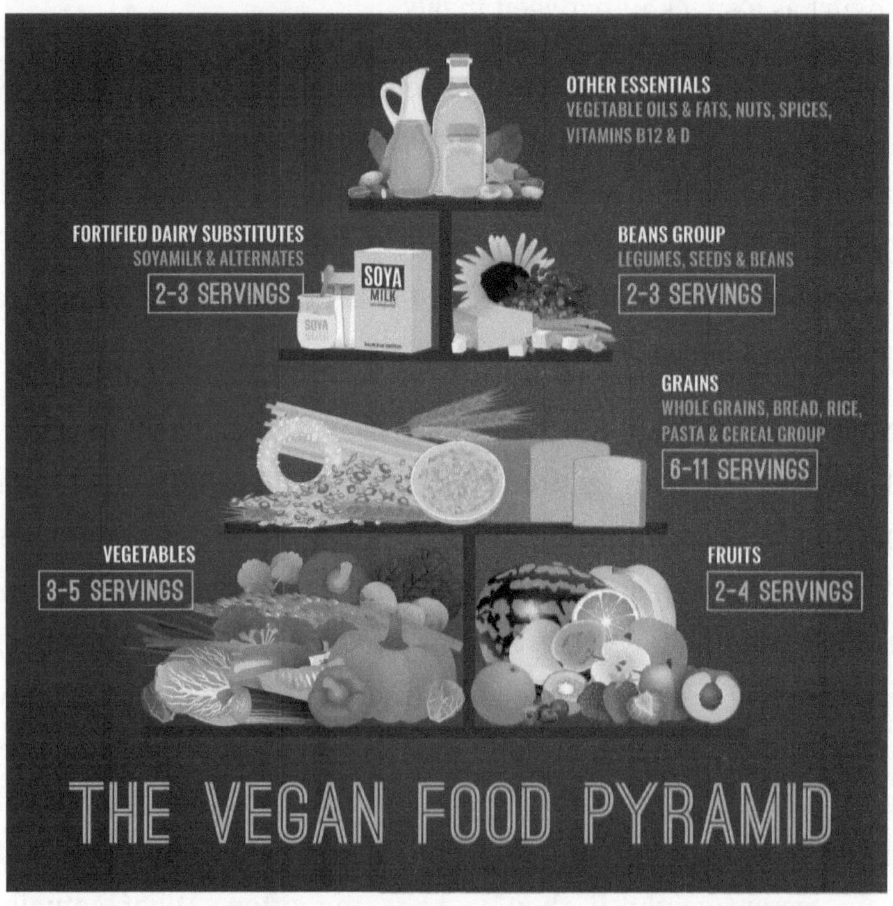

Veganism is on the rise, and if you are a vegan you need to know that you have options, HEALTHY options. Yes, not all vegan food is healthy for you. In fact, today's supermarkets are flooded with more junk food than healthy foods, even if it has the "vegan" stamp.

The problem isn't finding variety and nutrition in the vegan diet, even though many people seem to think that's the main problem. It's finding products that aren't loaded with sugar and fat. Why are so many vegan alternatives like that? Just think about all the vegan "meats" and various products that are designed to taste like actual bacon and pork sausage, for example. These food items contain pretty much everything you should avoid. So, before we climb the vegan pyramid, make sure you check nutritional values and ingredients on the label. The vegan diet trend made many food corporations see nothing but dollar signs, so they pushed a lot of unhealthy products.

With that out of the way, you can follow a healthy vegan food diet without missing any nutrients. Most vegans that are overweight, or lack something, are in that situation because they eat without being informed. This is where the vegan pyramid comes in without pushing you to memorize too much.

At the base of the pyramid, which will make up most of your diet, we find a variety of vegetables, berries, and other fruit. They should form the bulk of every meal. To maintain a balanced vegan diet, you should try to eat three servings of berries, and three servings of any other fruit on a daily basis. In addition, you should eat another three servings of vegetables. You can combine these servings as much as you like since there are so many types of fruits and veggies to choose from, and you can cook them in so many different ways. Just try to keep away from eating too much store-bought dry fruit because some manufacturers actually add sugar to it. After all, the fruits themselves are expensive, and sugar is cheap so it's common for producers to compensate and make the product heavier with added sugar. Additionally, dried fruit concentrates the sugars in fruit, so you can easily over-do your sugar consumption, even in the guise of healthy fruit. So, I recommend you only eat dried fruit in moderation.

Next, we have everything that is made with whole grains. As you can see grains are part of every diet. Carbs are commonly depicted as your enemy, however, whole grains contain essential vitamins and fiber, so you should eat around three servings of things like oats or quinoa.

Climbing the ladder, we have legumes and whole foods that contain healthy fats. This category includes mainly products that are rich in protein, such as kidney beans, black beans. This is also where tofu and tempeh is added to your list. You should consume three servings of these legumes, together with another three servings of fatty foods like nuts, seeds, and avocados. Remember, that no matter the diet you go for, the nutritional requirements stay the same. So, make sure to eat these healthy fats to avoid health problems caused by the lack of fat.

Finally, at the top we have the fatty foods (not to be confused with the healthy fatty foods like nuts). This is the category that mostly contains vegetable oils. So, if you are used to stir frying your vegetables often, or making salad dressing, you need to cut back on that habit. You shouldn't consume more than one serving a day, preferably even less. Sounds a bit daunting? Well, it doesn't have to be! Fortunately, in vegan dishes you can easily replace ingredients like olive oil, with water or vegetable stock. Sure, your food might not be crunchy, but the yummy flavors will still be there. At least you will significantly cut back on calories.

Now, since this is a vegan diet, you will have to supplement certain nutritions that you can't find naturally in plant-based foods. For instance, B12 supplements should be taken daily. In addition, you might have to take iron if you don't eat iron-rich vegetables like spinach. Lastly, Omega-3 also needs to be supplemented, but it can be done through food. All you need to do is add a couple of tablespoons of flax seeds or chia seeds to your meals. Fish isn't the only source of Omega-3 fatty acids. If you don't like those seeds though, the alternative is taking a supplement made out of algaes that also contain Omega-3s.

A healthy vegan diet is just as possible as any other. You won't lack nutrients as long as you eat smart and you add a lot of variety to your daily eating habits. Moreover, stay away from heavily processed vegan foods advertised by the big companies, and stick to the basics.

The Paleo Pyramid

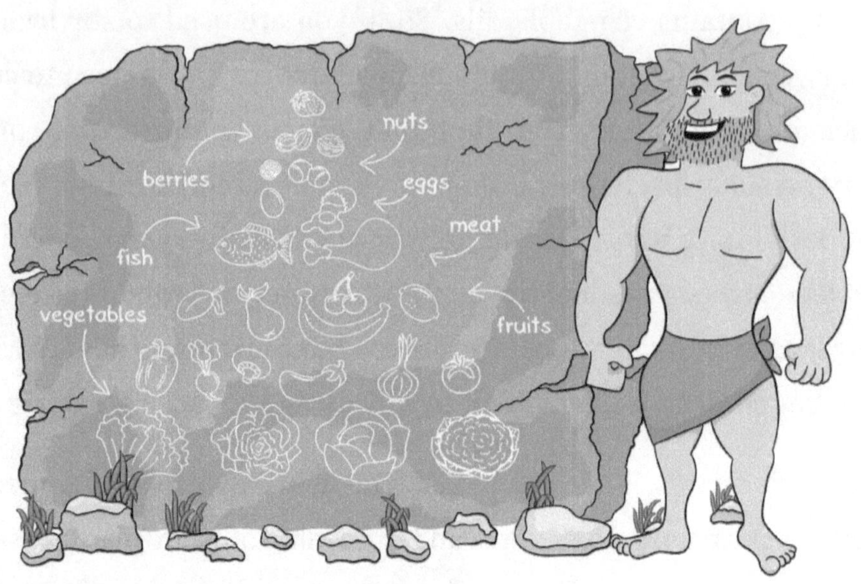

The Paleo diet became a huge hit in the 2000s when more and more people started realizing the risks behind heavily processed foods. Since this is the "caveman" diet, it focuses on foods that nature provides without any, or much, intervention from man.

During the paleolithic era, humans ate whatever they could hunt or gather. Farming wasn't a thing yet, so our ancestors simply ate whatever meat, fish, fruits, and vegetables they could find. The paleo pyramid is built to represent their diet. While the historical accuracy of it's still questioned because we can't know for certain what the ancient man ate, the diet will eliminate all processed foods that we all got used to eating on a regular basis, sometimes without even knowing.

The idea behind the diet is to create meals that are rich in low-starch vegetables, which means no products such as rice and corn because farming didn't appear yet in the paleolithic period. The diet is also rich in healthy fats, mostly from nuts, and fruit like avocados. Another key aspect of the diet is consuming protein from animals that have been raised naturally, on grass mostly. Keep in mind that animals are farmed intensely nowadays in order to keep up with the demand and to maintain low prices. This means that animals are rarely raised on open pastures.

The paleo pyramid serves as a guide for this diet, however, it isn't an exact science because we can only assume what people ate back then. Fortunately, this guide works the same as all the other pyramids. The foods at the bottom should be eaten often, while the foods closer to the top should be eaten occasionally. One thing to keep in mind though, is that serving sizes aren't precise. They depend on your particular dietary requirements. Therefore, you should keep a goal in mind. Do you need to lose weight? Do you want to build muscle mass? Depending on these answers, you can use the paleo pyramid to prepare your diet. If you aren't sure and you want to play safe however, you should probably speak to a nutritionist or dietician to fully understand the paleo serving sizes you should aim for.

With that being said, at the base of the paleo pyramid we have plants. Lots of plants! Again, they have to be non-starchy. So, nothing like grains and potatoes. The bulk of your meals should be formed by spinach, broccoli, peppers, radishes, asparagus, cauliflower, and so on. The more leafy greens and juicy vegetables you eat, the better. Because of the low calorie count in non-starchy vegetables, you can have your fill and easily eat up to three servings for every meal.

Next up we have proteins, and plenty of them. Never forget proteins, whether you choose a vegan diet or a paleo diet. This pyramid recommends eggs, steaks, bacon, and organs like iron-rich livers. All of these animal products should come from grass-fed animals only, not just due to the idea behind the paleolithic diet, but also because they are of higher quality, more nutritious. As a bonus, a grass-fed animal also leads a much better life than one that is stuck in a warehouse throughout the year. Regarding servings, you can go for anywhere between three to six daily.

In the middle of the pyramid we have fats, and rich foods in general. These meals focus on nutritious foods that are also very healthy for your stomach and the entire digestive system. Think of kefir, and other fermented products, nuts, and avocados. As a bonus, you can also go for the bone broth and get the full caveman experience! That might be a joke, probably a bad one, but bone broths are in fact very healthy and nutritious because they are rich in protein, healthy fats, and minerals like calcium and magnesium. Plus, this way you make sure you use every part of the animal and waste nothing. Our ancestors held a deep respect for nature and used every part of the animal. Just aim for one serving per meal and your body will be nourished.

If you're an athlete, or you work out a lot, you have the option to consume natural sugars from honey, maple syrup, and various sugary fruits. Just eat them sparingly depending on how active you are. In addition, you can occasionally reward yourself with dark chocolate, wine, or mead, since they can be considered paleo. Just make sure you don't overdo it. For instance, having two squares of non-sugary chocolate per day is perfectly fine.

Please Consult Your Doctor

If you have any health problems or particular dietary restrictions, you should consult your doctor. Food affects your body directly. Various products can worsen an illness or make you sick. For instance, if you're suffering from diabetes, you will obviously have some restrictions and you can't follow these pyramid guides precisely. In other cases, people get sick from milk or other dairy products, or they have various allergies to nuts or gluten. So, if you're aware of such medical problems, consult your doctor before you get started. He or she can also direct you to a nutritionist or dietician who is made aware of your restrictions and health issues.

Summary

Still not 100% sure where to start? No problem! Just start by looking at which goals you want to achieve. Based on the goal, and your dietary preference, you can choose the diet. The pyramid guides we discussed in this chapter are simple guidelines and nothing more. They aren't a magic solution to living healthy and they aren't particularly designed to promote weight loss, or gain, or anything else. The purpose of these pyramids is to inform you on how to get the nutrients you need to live a healthy life. The rest is up to you. So, figure out your goals and what you need in order to achieve them.

Chapter 3: Nutrition and Weight Loss Myths

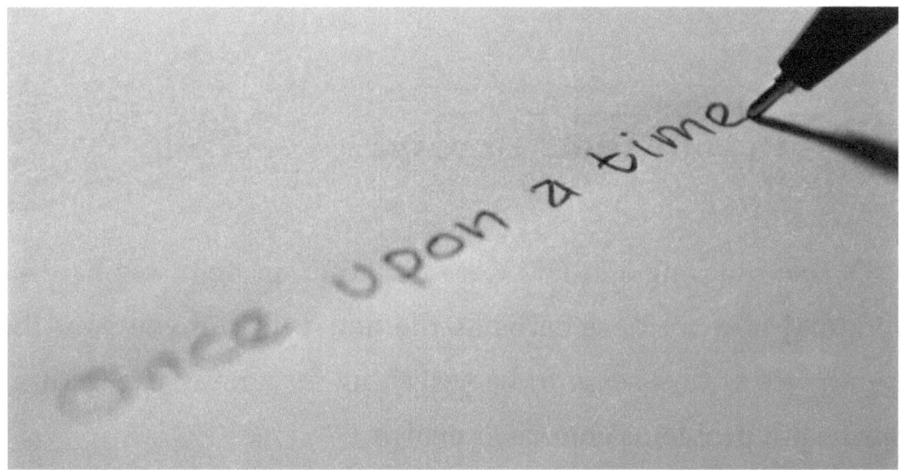

Misconceptions and myths about eating healthy and staying in shape should've disappeared with Google, right? Wrong, unfortunately. Even though we have all this information available and it's so easy to learn pretty much anything, we still fall for misinformation and made up fairytales. The digital age made our access to information much easier, but the stories that used to be spread by your gossipy aunt simply switched from the word of mouth to Facebook and other social media channels. With today's media bombardment, even the stories you hear from official sources are sometimes unverified or unconfirmed. So, your only real option is to read the original medical studies to learn the truth, and let's face it, nobody really wants to do that.

With that being said, in this chapter we are going to debunk the most common myths around nutrition and weight loss. In each section we will explore the misconceptions and learn the truth without digging too deep into stone-cold theory. After all, that's why you're reading this book instead of research papers from Harvard.

Carbs in your Diet? Heresy!

Let's see, not long ago fats were evil, then protein was bad for you, and now we have carbs as the new evil. Did you spot the trend? We always seem to be searching for a new scapegoat as our health problems change or evolve.

In the case of carbs, a lot of people think that the glycemic index, or even the insulin index, allows them to rank foods by how healthy or unhealthy they are. They believe that a low glycemic diet will keep them healthier, but in reality, there's almost no difference even among diabetics. The advantage given by a low glycemic diet is so slight that in reality it won't have any noticeable positive effects over your metabolism. In fact, foods with a low glycemic index won't even offer you any improvement over your glycemic control (PubMed, 2018).

In addition, several studies were done to see if there's a significant difference in weight loss when going through a low carb, high carb, or keto diet. All of these diets had the same result in the end, since they were all designed to lead to weight loss, even though the food items differed (PubMed, 2013).

Eating fewer carbs might help you personally, or maybe make your diet easier, since most carb rich foods are higher in calories and lower in certain nutrients. However, that doesn't mean you should eliminate carbs. You can consume them normally, while you make other adjustments in your diet. So, if you're trying to lose weight, just make sure your body gets all of the nutrients it needs and you stay at a caloric deficit. In other words, if you don't overdo it, there's nothing unhealthy about consuming carbs.

Protein Isn't Good for You

Yes, this is a myth. You absolutely need protein, even if you're a vegan. However, this is a popular misconception similar to the one about carbs and fats (we'll get to this one next). So why do people think protein is harmful? Apparently, for various reasons, some of them think that protein consumption can lead to damaged bones... and kidneys. Huh?

The first theory about bones most likely stems because of a few theories about high protein diets resulting in a high content of calcium in urine. This led some people to believe that the heightened acidity levels caused by too much protein had to be combated by calcium, which would be drawn from the bones. As a result, some believe that if they eat too much protein, their bones will weaken. None of this is true.

The reason why calcium appeared in urine in people consuming lots of protein is because the source of the protein was mostly dairy products. When you eat a lot of dairy, which is rich in calcium, you pee it out. The reality is that when you eat a lot of protein, your body actually absorbs more calcium than usual, which is a good thing. Low protein diets are in fact connected to a higher risk of bone fractures, particularly hip fractures (PubMed, 2017).

The way it works is that when you eat protein, calcium is absorbed better instead of ending up in your feces. However, your body notices later that it doesn't need all that calcium, so it proceeds to eliminate it through your urine. That's all there is to it. So, protein is actually very good for your body and your bones.

The other myth mentioned is the one about kidney damage, which is also untrue. The idea is that when you eat a lot of protein, your kidneys seem to work harder to filter out the bad stuff. Some people think that if the kidneys increase their filtration rate, they're working too hard and they will suffer damage. Fortunately, there's no evidence that proves high protein consumption can cause that. This particular study (PubMed, 2018) shows that all of this is a myth.

In conclusion, stick to consuming regular amounts of protein without worrying about these stories that are sometimes circulating through social media. Protein is necessary, it's good for you, and your bones and muscles.

Fat Is what Makes You Fat (Nope)

We've all heard this tired old myth. No, eating fats does NOT make you fat by itself. If you follow a balanced diet and eat the amount of calories you should for your body weight, sex, age, and fitness level, then it really doesn't matter if you eat a moderate amount of fat or no fat. In fact, eliminating fat entirely is dangerous! Your body needs healthy fats, like omega-3 and omega-6 to keep you in good shape. Another fat-related myth is the one about saturated fat being what causes cardiovascular diseases. No, that type of fat isn't the main factor behind those health problems.

In reality, only trans fats are proven to be bad for your health (NAP, 2005). This is true for both natural trans fats, as well as the manufactured ones. However, if you consume them only from natural sources, the quantities are too small to actually matter. Just avoid industrially produced cookies, pastries, and other trans fat rich foods that are heavily processed.

Fortunately, the FDA effectively banned trans fats in 2018, and any of the products using trans fats were given until 2019 to phase them out. (FDA, 2018). However, you can probably still find products containing trans fats as of the writing of this book (2020). So, make sure you check the labels, just in case.

In conclusion, low fat diets won't help you get in shape if you're eating more calories than you should. The best thing to do is to balance your diet to get all the nutrients you need, such as omega-3 fatty acids. We will talk more about fats in a later chapter because this is an important topic that is key to a healthy nutrition and lifestyle.

Detoxing? Oh No You Don't!

Going through detox diets, or cleansing diets, is probably the biggest trend nowadays and it's all nonsense and quackery. If you "detox" yourself by drinking nothing but plant juices, with supplements on top, you need to stop... yesterday. This may sound harsh, perhaps even offensive if you're into "detoxing", but this is something that can put you in danger. Just ask your doctor or any real medical professional about this practice if you don't believe me.

So, what is this detox trend anyway? Firstly, the term "detox" is medically used only when someone is undergoing recovery from addictive substances, such as alcohol and heroine. Obviously, in this case we aren't talking about that scenario. In the past decade, a new trend appeared, pushing for cleansing our bodies in a healthy way. The general idea is that we can lose weight, focus better, and gain more energy by eliminating all the toxins that gather in the system. Take note that in this case the word toxin is used, by those who promote detoxing, as a buzzword to portray some nefarious substances inside you.

The truth is that if we truly have some nasty substances in our bodies, we would certainly feel it over time. Just think about mercury poisoning, asbestos, cyanide, alcohol, etc. If you are exposed to a real toxic substance, no broccoli juice is going to help with anything. Keep in mind that the only exception here would be ingesting activated charcoal because that can help you if you ate something that was poisonous. Whatever toxin you consume, like alcohol, will either damage you, or it will be filtered by your body's real detox system, which consists of a number of organs. That's right, your body comes fully equipped with toxin filtration systems! Otherwise the human species would've died out a long time ago.

It's true that we are exposed to various toxins quite often, however, they are handled by our kidneys, liver, and intestines, not our diet. For instance, the liver is in charge of producing the enzymes that break down most of the toxic metals and drugs so that you can eliminate them. Without a liver, you can no longer flush out many such harmful toxins no matter what you do.

Your blood also gathers toxins over time and this is where your kidney comes in to save the day. The main purpose of your kidneys is to filter out your blood and eliminate the toxins your body produces as byproducts, such as lactic acid and urea. Once these substances are filtered, you simply pee them out. Living without kidneys is possible as you surely heard, but it's far from a pleasant experience. People with no kidneys have to go onto a program of dialysis, usually several times a week, in order to filter all the bad stuff in their blood. Without that procedure, the toxic substances would end up killing them.

The detox trend however focuses on the digestive system. Those who keep pushing this idea, that if you drink plenty of juices, all the bad stuff in your intestines will be flushed out. The problem with this practice is that you don't just eliminate what's bad. You also get rid of the intestinal flora that is vital for maintaining a healthy digestive system. Do you remember taking antibiotics and the doctor recommending you something to protect your intestinal flora or your guts in general? That's because antibiotics kill all bacteria, including the friendly kind that lives inside you to keep you healthy. Once our little friends die off, the bad guys are free to move in and cause an infectious form of diarrhea, or worse.

Through so-called detoxing, and even colon cleansing, you won't benefit from anything other than putting yourself at risk. If you would truly need to undergo a form of medical detoxing, you would already feel sick and experience some nasty symptoms. The human body can deal with many toxic substances found all around us on its own. By going on a liquid diet for a few days, or some extreme form of fasting, you will just weaken your body. In fact, by going through such extremes you might eliminate certain nutrients that your detoxing organs require to properly function at peak performance. So please don't put yourself in danger, read more about how your body works from a medical standpoint, and even talk to a doctor if you are still not convinced or unsure.

This may lead you to another question. Why do certain people feel so good after going through a period of detoxing? The answer to that is pretty simple. Nowadays, we are aware of many things that harm us, and we want to treat our mortal bodies like a temple. We are used to snacking, eating junk food, buying frozen pizzas and other heavily processed stuff that's terrible for us. Therefore, when we stop eating all of that junk for a week, we start not just feeling better, but also feeling better about ourselves.

So, if you truly want to be as free of toxins as possible, then here's some advice that is suggested by medical sources (Harvard Health Publishing, 2008). Eat a healthy, balanced diet to get all the nutrients you need, hydrate yourself with pure water, exercise every day, sleep well, and don't forget to get yourself checked up on a regular basis to be safe. That's it! If you do that, you can leave everything else to your body, which is a very sophisticated piece of machinery, so handle it with care.

Lose the Bread to Lose Weight

Ah, the good ol' "all you need to do is stop eating bread and you'll have the body of your dreams" myth. Actually, there are two arguments related to bread. First, some people think that bread makes them fat. Second, there are those who think that gluten is bad and since bread contains it, we should stop eating it.

The first myth is actually understandable since bread is rich in calories. It's very easy to eat too much of it, especially because we tend to eat it with things like butter, Nutella, and cheese. These foods and condiments are highly dense in calories, so you can overeat your entire calorie allowance for the day during breakfast if you aren't careful. However, this isn't the bread's fault. Just because it's high in calories doesn't mean it's making you fat. As with everything else, you should eat bread in moderation. It can be included in a healthy diet by making sure you don't go over your calorie limit and just eat a slice of toast, not five.

The second myth is about gluten and how it's dangerous for everyone to consume. Yes, gluten can be dangerous to those with celiac disease (less than 1% of the population), an autoimmune condition (PubMed, 2015). The same study estimates that around 6.5% are just sensitive to gluten but they can tolerate it. That being said, if you are one of these people, cut the bread out of your diet. If you think you might be intolerant, get a diagnosis to make sure it's not something else. Otherwise, feel free to eat bread because gluten is just a protein. Yes, it's a protein, not a type of carbohydrate or something toxic to our health like some people mistakenly believe.

Finally, we have the white bread versus whole wheat bread argument. You've probably been hearing this from the media for years how whole wheat bread is far healthier than white bread. The idea is that whole wheat bread offers roughly the same amount of calories, but it has a lower glycemic index (we discussed this earlier). In addition, it also has a higher fiber content. This is all true, but what you weren't told is that the difference in fiber and nutrient content is so low that it doesn't even matter. There are fruits and veggies with more fiber and nutrients than whole wheat bread. So, don't try to get your daily fiber from bread or you are going to eat way too much of it.

Feel free to eat any bread you like, as long as you calculate your calorie and nutrient intake. It can easily be incorporated in your diet and it doesn't matter if it's white, brown, graham, whole wheat and so on. And if you think gluten is causing you some issues, go have a talk with your doctor. You shouldn't diagnose yourself.

We Need Supplements

The supplement industry continues to grow and advertise using a number of buzzwords like "clinically proven" in order to sell vitamins to those who most likely don't even need them. By the way, that label is just a sales pitch that can mean anything and it doesn't even require any evidence to back it up.

Nutrition supplements aren't bad for you and they can help if your diet doesn't provide you with something. For instance, if you're low on iron, you can take an iron supplement and see some improvements. The problem is that a myth was spread that made many people believe that the quality of food is now lower than it used to be decades ago, due to industrialization.

Supplements have their use, but if your diet supplies you with everything you need, there's no point in spending any money on vitamin pills. Your body can only absorb so much. Any mineral, vitamin, or protein you consume in addition to what a normal human being can process, will end up in your pee or feces. So, when you have a proper diet, all you get from multivitamins is expensive pee.

What you should do is look at your diet, see if you are getting all the macro and micronutrients you need. You can also get occasionally tested and check out all the nutrient levels in your system. If something is missing, you can find the food that provides you with what you need. Or, take a supplement in that case.

Supplements are useful and you can benefit from them, but their purpose is to fill in gaps in your diet, not replace healthy foods.

Eat Clean, Eat Raw, Be Healthy

This isn't necessarily a myth. It's a collection of several misconceptions. The first problem is that most people that follow this mantra don't agree on what eating clean means. Some believe in eating nothing but raw, organic foods. Some eliminate certain products, usually derived from animals, for various reasons. Others are only talking about pesticide and hormone-free foods. The only thing that brings all of the clean eaters together is the fact that they eliminate something from their diet.

So, let's tackle misconception number one: eating raw is good for you because you don't destroy all the nutrients. This is a myth, and eating raw isn't necessarily always good for you, because it depends on the food. The raw food gurus often even recommend drinking raw milk and eating raw eggs because that will preserve all the good nutrients inside. Well, raw milk is a terrible example because it often contains harmful bacteria. Even the peasants of old, before electricity, usually boiled or heated the milk before drinking it. As for eggs, your body will actually gain more protein from them when cooked than when raw (PubMed, 1999). Finally, even eating raw or cooked vegetables involves some kind of balance. For instance, if you cook veggies, you will reduce the amount of nitrate in them. Sure, this isn't good because that nitrate is important for blood pressure regulation. However, cooking them also eliminates the content of oxalate, which is a good thing. So, you can't say that eating raw everything is good for you, but it'sn't inherently bad either. You just need to pick your battles and form a balance.

Next, we have the idea that organic is the best. Nature = good, while artificial = bad. Makes sense, right? Well, there are quite a few scientific studies that tried to prove that, and they didn't manage to show that organic food leads to better health (Pubmed, 2012). This doesn't mean you shouldn't care about the type of food, but the problem is a complex one. For instance, even organic foods are grown using pesticides, though they are natural. However, some natural pesticides are just as bad for you as the synthetic ones, and sometimes even worse for the environment. So, eat organic food if you want and you can afford it, no problem, but please make sure to wash them and even peel them just the same.

Chicken Breast is All You Need to Lose Weight

This is one of the biggest myths when it comes to weight loss. A lot of people talk about eating nothing but boiled white meat and plain vegetables. Sure, you can lose weight this way since you can easily go into a calorie deficiency, however, you will not be healthy.

Losing weight this way is not recommended. This isn't a balanced diet at all and you will miss out on a great deal of nutrients. Chances are you will also fail to meet the recommended amount of protein you need to maintain your muscle mass. Take note that when you lose weight, you don't just burn fat. In order to compensate for the loss of nutrients and energy, the body starts eating away at your muscles as well as your fat stores.

Another problem with this method is that you will feel horrible during the diet. Your will to improve your lifestyle will be sapped, and you will constantly suffer from cravings. Plus, once you do lose your weight this way, you will probably go back to your previous diet that wasn't this boring. Once that happens, the pounds will come back to haunt you.

Don't starve yourself and don't deprive yourself from the healthy nutrients you need to function. Otherwise you will start losing focus, you will slow down at work, your memory can worse, you will no longer be able to be physically active and in the long term you can experience damaging health problems. Eat a varied diet, control the amount of calories you consume, exercise, drink water, and keep your weight off for good.

Summary

There are many myths and misconceptions about nutrition, eating healthy, and losing weight. Since food and diet are such hot topics nowadays, everyone is trying to take advantage of them in some way. Bloggers spread their own opinions, often uninformed and without any backing from scientific sources, companies prey on people with terms that don't mean what common sense tells you they mean, and so on. The bottom line is that you need to be skeptical about what you hear online from others, especially through social media, and stick to the basics.

Chapter 4: What to Eat

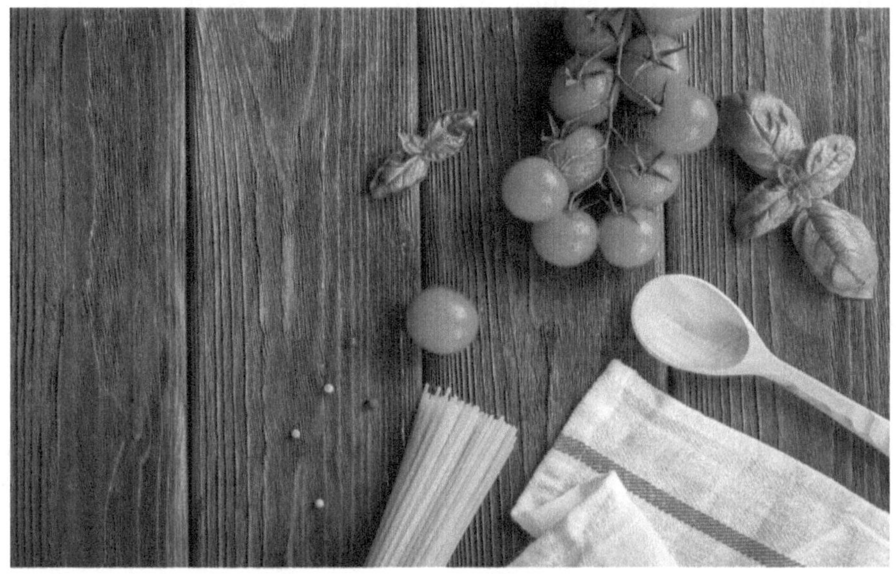

No matter which type of diet you choose, you will have to plan it in such a way to guarantee a balance between variety, nutrients, and the joy of eating.

So far, we mostly focused on pyramid guides. While they are useful and you should use them to get a rough idea about your daily diet, they don't offer a detailed picture. In this chapter, you will learn how to choose your healthy meals, how to plan them around your schedule. You will also learn how to optimize your shopping and prepare a weekly menu to get your started on your path to healthy nutrition.

Planning

This phase is essential. Establishing a routine is important in all aspects of your life, including eating. Eating healthy requires a certain degree of awareness. You should eat at regular times, especially if you normally don't. This can be tough, but you can train yourself. At the very least, you should go for what's considered "normal eating," namely planning breakfast, lunch, and dinner. Healthy snacks can also be added throughout the day.

Not eating for extended periods of time can have an influence over what you eat and how much. Remember the last time you went shopping on an empty stomach and instead of buying food for lunch, you bought three days worth of supplies? When you're really hungry, it's hard to measure how much food you should have for your meal. This can be dangerous and cause you to overeat.

Go back to one of the pyramid guides for the basic information so that you know what foods are available to you depending on your type of diet. First you need to make sure that all of your meals will contain plenty of nutrients from plant sources, like vegetables, fruits and grains. As mentioned earlier, these food items make the bulk of most diets because they are lower in calories and fats, but higher in nutrients. Next, you can pick your protein sources, just avoid the ones that have too much fat. Focus on variety! Don't be afraid to try something new. You can easily make a seemingly boring healthy diet fun and exciting. Just don't forget that sweets and fats are treats, so before you eat any processed food, read the label to see how many calories you'll get.

Breakfast's Ready!

Busy schedule? Work starts at odd hours? All it takes is a few minutes and a little bit of discipline and you will never skip breakfast again. Now, breakfast skipping isn't as bad as you think, as long as you're an average person with no serious health conditions. Some people think that skipping breakfast will mess with their metabolism, but that isn't the case. The real issue is that by skipping the first meal of the day, you will be less energetic than you could be. Naturally, this might not be an issue for you since we're all different. But a lot of people perform better after breaking fast in the morning, and they have better portion control throughout the day because they won't feel the need to eat a horse.

Fortunately, having a healthy breakfast can take a few minutes. Not having time because of work or a busy schedule is just an excuse.

The first thing you can do if you're busy is start eating cereal. This cold breakfast can be highly nutritious, doesn't require cooking skills, and you can eat it in no time. But there are so many breakfast cereals out there and not all of them are created equal.

Always read the label! Here's why. A one cup serving of All-Bran, for example, contains as little as 160 calories. Granola, in the same quantity, can contain up to 450 calories. Massive difference! Some cereals contain a lot of sugar in order to make them more exciting. You need to keep away from these. They aren't that nutritious, and you end up eating a lot of calories without gaining much in return. That's a really bad deal. So, check the label, choose a low-calorie cereal (keep your breakfast at or under 300 calories) and pay attention to the nutrients as well. Fortunately, most cereal brands these days are fortified with vitamins and minerals, and just by having a serving for breakfast you can get up to around 25% of your daily nutrient requirements.

If you aren't crazy about cereal, you don't have to eat it every single day. You can replace it with a whole wheat bagel, one or two teaspoons of peanut butter, and one banana. If you also add a glass for low fat milk to this breakfast, you should still be below 400 calories which is ok.

Another option is having an eggcellent breakfast. You can eat 2 whole eggs, once or twice a week. They are highly nutritious and filling. The reason why you shouldn't eat more than that is that the cholesterol levels are quite high in the egg yolk. So, try to stick to eating fewer than five eggs per week. Optionally, you could use one whole egg, plus two egg whites to make a healthier breakfast.

As you can see there are quite a few options, and all of these are inspired from the food groups described in the food pyramid.

Now let's say you REALLY don't have time for breakfast at home, so you tend to eat out. That's ok, you can still eat out, but you need to be even more careful. Calories hide in places you don't expect, and restaurants and cafes tend to add quite a bit of extra fats and sugars into their products to make them taste better. So, stick to the basics, like cereals, bagels, fruits, and yogurt. Doesn't sound like a very interesting eat-out, but you need to make sacrifices for your health sometimes. So, try to replace the unhealthier things you eat out. For instance, you can switch from a bran muffin to an English muffin which is a lot lower in calories. If you like granola, switch to bran cereals. Instead of a doughnut, have a bagel. You get the idea.

Lunch Time

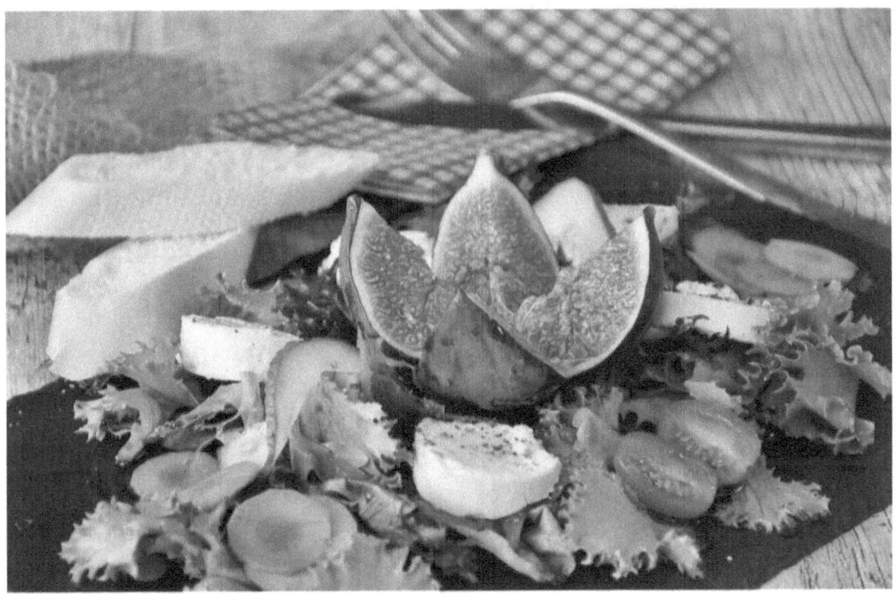

This is a meal that many people eat in a restaurant, cafeteria, or the company break room. This makes it hard for some to eat healthy because they're in a rush, in the middle of their working hours, so they just go to eat whatever is accessible and affordable to their budget.

Lunch is important because it's one of the big meals that keeps you going throughout your busy day. This is why you should follow the same rules as before. Eat well but eat healthy. Pay attention to the nutrients, and especially the bad things that come with a hearty lunch, such as too much saturated fat. Since this meal is usually bigger than breakfast, this is when you should eat the most fruit, vegetables, and grains. All of these food groups are packed with vitamins, minerals, and energy to keep you going. After all, you don't want to lose focus on the job and slip up. A healthy diet can help prevent that.

It's also worth mentioning that you don't have to eat out during your lunch hours. Eating at a restaurant or cafeteria is difficult because you can't always judge the amount of calories your meal will contain. And even if you can, you'll have trouble finding out the fat content, carb content, and so on. The solution is to pack something from home. This might not be fun and it may take some preparation skills, but you will save a lot of money in the long run, plus you will eat precisely the way you want to eat.

All you need to do is plan your meals. Look towards the pyramids for guidance, and decide accordingly. Make sure all the major food groups will be present in your lunch and that you will consume enough calories. After all, this meal is going to keep you going until dinner time (with a little help from some healthy snacks). If you don't have a balanced lunch, you will most likely end up really hungry before dinner time and eat too much.

Since a lot of people aren't too happy with bringing a lunch box every day, the key to adjusting to this lifestyle is once again variety. Let's face it, even when we try to lose weight, gain muscle, or just eat healthy, we try to make our meals fun. People love food. Food makes us happy, and there's no reason to be miserable when eating. You can eat healthy and still have fun. So, here are some simple ideas:

1. For grains, don't always opt for the same plain, boring, bread sandwich. Learn to use tortilla wraps, or flatbread, lettuce or even rice cakes. You can also replace this with a salad that contains some healthy grains and seeds.

2. As for fruit, eat fresh! Don't go for sugary fruit salads you often find in stores. Just pack your favorite fruit. They come in such a variety that every day you can eat something different. Try new things as well, anything that's exotic, to keep it interesting.

3. Don't forget the veggies! Vegetables make up most of any diet, so feel free to go wild. Eat raw carrots, spinach, tomatos, chilli pepper, and anything you like. Prepare salads or you can even cook soup! You don't have to carry the liquid if it isn't practical, but you can still take out the cooked veggies and have them as a side dish. You can also stir-fry your vegetables, but either use a very small amount of oil, or vegetable stock. Another option is veggies juice along with your meal.

4. Add some low-fat dairy products to the mix. One day you can have yogurt, another you can drink some milk, or even eat some cheese. Just don't overdo it because dairy products are quite fatty and high in calories.

5. Finally, you can have some meat, unless you're a vegan of course. The idea is to have a nice source of protein, which doesn't have to be meat. It can be any type of bean or nuts. However, if you're used to having meat as the main course, you might have some issues adjusting. Meat should be part of your diet, but not the central part. In order to cut back, replace some of it with various veggies and fruits. There are plenty of protein sources, so start experimenting while paying attention to calories, fat content, and other nutrients.

Taking food to work with you is a great option, but you will still want to occasionally eat out. When doing so, you should follow all the guidelines we established earlier, however, there are two more bits of useful advice.

Restaurants and fast food places love adding healthy sounding names to some of their salads and burgers. They also use the word "diet" occasionally and it doesn't really mean what you think it means. Sure, the product may have fewer calories than the original version, but it can still be worth 1000 calories or any other amount. In addition, salads can easily trick you. When you eat out you should stick to simple salads. Those tasty dressings they add are loaded with fat and sugars, thus increasing the calorie count of a salad to that of a burger. Speaking of burgers, you should avoid them entirely, unless you plan some kind of cheat day once in two weeks or so. To give you an example, a burger with "double" or "deluxe" in its name can go way over 1000 calories. That's half of your daily calorie intake in one single burger! Let's not even think about the nutrients and the quality of ingredients. It's better to make them yourself at home because that way you'll know what ingredients you should use in order to eat according to your diet plan.

What's for Dinner?

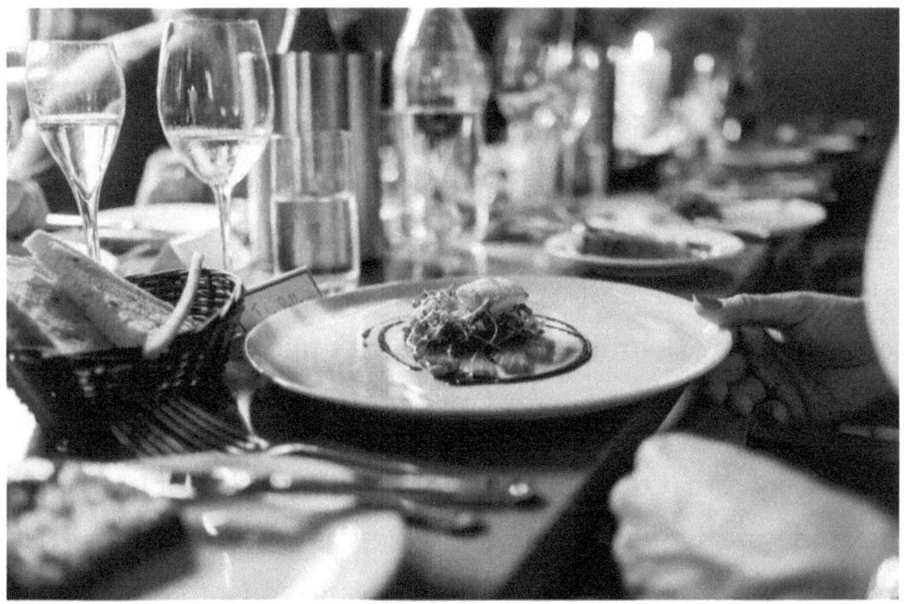

This is an important meal because this is often the time to socialize, whether it's with family, friends or both. Unfortunately, many people have other concerns around dinner time, such as house work, extra duties from the office, a child's school play, and so on. We are so busy nowadays that it can seem impossible to find the time to prepare a proper dinner. However, even if you get overwhelmed sometimes, you can still take control of the situation with a little bit of planning. Eating healthy when busy is a skill, but with time and practice, you'll be an expert in no time.

The first thing you need to do is make time. You rolled your eyes a bit, didn't you? That's alright, perfectly normal reaction to such an obvious "solution." People often use the lack of time as an excuse, but the truth is that most people suck at planning their precious time. Do you think famous bodybuilders like Arnold Schwarzenegger stopped paying attention to diet and workouts because they were travelling or working? No! If they have to go to work at 7, they find time to exercise at 6. Take a look at your schedule. Put it on paper, including all your free time and duties outside of work. This way you will notice windows of opportunity. You will see ways to combine some of your responsibilities in order to free up some time. Five minutes here, ten minutes there, and bam! You have time for dinner.

Once you get that out of the way, you can go to the fun part and make the magic happen. Again, variety is key! You should take something from each major food group and add it to your dinner. Eat more vegetables, together with small amounts of low-fat meats and dairy products. Experiment with foods from other cultures to keep things interesting. In other parts of the world people barely eat any meat, so they come up with mind blowing recipes based on fruits and veggies alone. You'll soon realize that cooking isn't some talent. It's just a skill that allows you to use your imagination and experiment.

For dinner, you want an explosion of vitamins, minerals, and fiber. Look at the large variety of breads, like pumpernickel or rye. Or look at pasta, which comes in so many forms, and you can cook a dish focused around spinach, or tomatoes. Replace red meat with fish, or at least poultry. Be adventurous and try game birds instead of the usual turkey and chicken. Finally, finish your dinner with some fresh fruit and low-fat cheese. Or go for sherbet! A glass of wine is also acceptable.

Dinners don't have to take you a long time to cook. Stick to the basics if you don't have time. Cook once when you actually have time, but cook in higher quantities. Then you'll have food for the next day as well. Or you can even freeze a few portions for those evenings when you truly have no time to cook or you're too tired to think about food. Just don't skip on this meal.

Eating out is another option if you enjoy doing that and it's in your budget. However, due to the issues with restaurant food not being all that healthy, you'll need to do some research. Yes, there are places where you can find food that suits your diet. You just need to find them. Start searching for a restaurant that serves a wide array of vegetable and fruit dishes that aren't cooked with added fats. Most decent places will list the details you need to know. Once you find an adequate restaurant (doesn't have to be perfect), you can employ other methods to make sure you eat healthy:

1. Ask the chef to bake or broil the menu item that is listed as fried. The restaurant should be able to accommodate you and this simple change will already reduce the amount of fat and calories you consume.
2. If you'd like to order a salad, ask them to serve the dressing on the side. This way you have control over how much you eat since dressings are high in fat. In addition, you could ask them to replace the fatty dressing with a diet-friendly one.
3. Order small or prepare to take leftovers home with you. Avoid large servings of meals that are described as "jumbo" or anything similar.
4. Try not to drink more than two drinks. If you eat out on a daily basis, you should stick to one drink. Alcoholic beverages aren't free of calories. For instance, a regular beer can have upwards of 150 calories.

As you can see, you have plenty of options. Eating healthy is a choice, as well as sticking to your nutritious diet. So, make sure you develop a routine and keep your meals interesting. Healthy food doesn't have to be boring.

Shopping Correctly

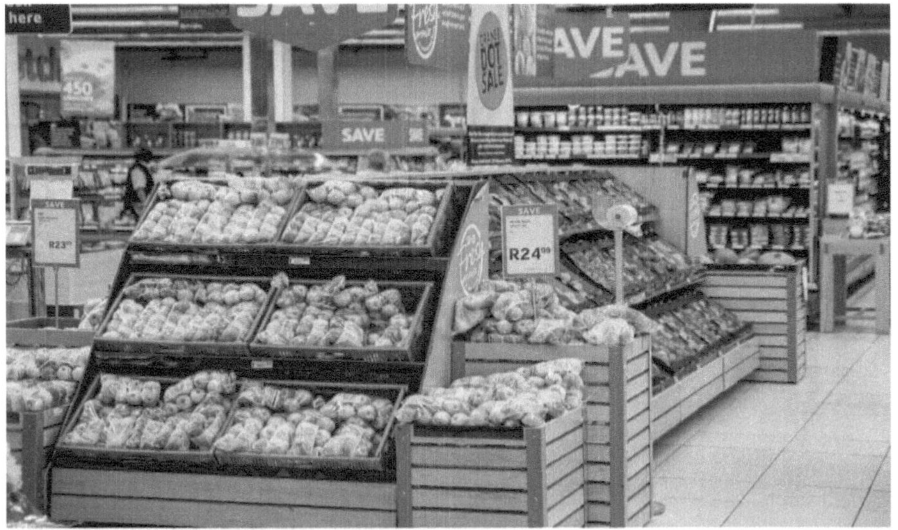

Don't you just hate it when you go shopping, you're determined to eat healthy, but then you see your favorite food or dessert? Don't punish yourself. That happens to all of us. All you need to do is plan a bit better, and take a few precautionary measures to avoid the temptation. Here's how you can improve your shopping experience and support your healthy habits:

1. Start by preparing a list. We like to think that we can remember what we need, but just think about all those times you went to the store to buy one specific item, but you ended up buying a bunch of other things except what you went for in the first place. This is why you need a clear list. It helps you save time and it tells you where to go. The more you wander aimlessly through a store, the more distractions and temptations you will have to face.

2. Don't go shopping on an empty stomach. This is probably the worst thing you can do. When you go hungry to the store, you end up buying a lot more food than you need and you are more likely to give into temptations. So, make sure you eat something before heading to the store. It doesn't have to be a meal. A snack is often all you need to curb your appetite for a while.

3. Be careful with special deals. Stores now that people are attracted to good bargains, like a 50% discount. Most of us care about our budget and when we see such a deal, we just go for it because it's too hard to pass on. So, when you go shopping, focus on your healthy diet and don't buy on impulse. If you don't usually eat pasta because of your diet, don't buy a pack of spaghetti, even if it's almost free. The temptation can be quite powerful, so just buy what you need. Less is more.

Finally, when you purchase a product, you need to pay attention to the label. A lot of people aren't even aware of how much they eat because they don't know how to read it or they don't really care. It's easy to say, "I don't eat much but I'm still gaining weight, it must be because of my hormones." A lot of people just don't realize how many calories flour or peanut butter have, for example. Plenty of us like to eat peanut butter jelly sandwiches, and multiple servings because we can't be satisfied by just one. This is how they end up eating half of their daily calorie allowance in one small meal that mostly contains carbs and fats.

How to Read a Product Label

These labels can be intimidating to some because they contain a lot of information, however, we'll pick this apart so that it's easier to understand.

The first thing the label shows is the serving size. Not every food is created equal, so a serving size of peanut butter won't weigh the same as a broiled chicken breast serving. The information on the label is based on the declared serving size, thus allowing you to make easier comparisons with other products. It doesn't take that long to take 3 competing products off the shelf and compare the nutrient and calorie values.

Once the serving is established, the labels should also specify how many servings there are in total, along with the caloric value of a single serving. The number of calories is very important, especially when you're trying to lose weight or maintain your current level. Next, you'll see a table with all the nutrients like fat, sodium, fiber, vitamin A, vitamin C, protein, magnesium, and so on. All of these are represented by two numbers, quantity, and the percent daily value. The quantity is normally listed in grams or milligrams, but what we're really interested in is the percent value. This number tells us what percentage of the daily requirement is provided by one serving. So, if, for instance, a serving of something says it provides 100% Calcium, that means it contains the amount of calcium you should consume in a day.

That's it. There's more information like calories from fat, or calories per gram, but it's enough to guide yourself by nutrient values and total calories per serving.

Daily Menus

In this section, I have a few examples of how your daily menus can look like. You don't have to eat these specific food items though. The purpose of this part is to guide you on how to plan your meals by measuring the amounts of nutrients and calories you need.

First, you need to determine your goals and analyze your current lifestyle. We discussed earlier in the book that a physically active person can eat more than someone who leads a sedentary life. In these examples we are going to assume you are a fairly balanced person that is only moderately active (30 minutes of daily physical activity). This means that our goal is to construct a menu worth a maximum of 2000 calories.

Next, we need to calculate how much fat our food will contain. The general rule is that a third of the calories can and should come from fat. Since fat is very rich, this means that we should consume less than 60 grams of fat throughout a normal day. Keep in mind that not all fat is created equal, so we should pay attention to saturated fat too (under 15 grams).

Fiber should be maintained at around 30 grams each day to meet the normal requirements. Finally, we have sodium, which matters because consuming too much of it can cause bad side effects like high blood pressure, and bloating. Don't consume more than around 2300 milligrams per day, but at least 500 milligrams, more if you're physically active.

As for the food groups, use the aforementioned pyramids to guide depending on which diet you choose. Following these guidelines, you can design any meal you like and control what you eat. With that being said, here are a few menus to get you started!

Example 1

Start your day with a balanced breakfast. You can have two whole wheat pancakes, with half a cup of your favorite fruit sauce. Just make sure it doesn't contain any added sugar. The fruit it's made from contains more than enough. Along with the pancakes you can also have a cup of nonfat or low-fat yogurt. Drink coffee or tea with your breakfast. Just take note that you should avoid putting any sugar or cream in these beverages. Without these additions, they basically contain no calories so you can drink as much as you want. The calories come from the sugar, cream, milk, etc.

For lunch, you can go for a healthy Caesar salad. Just make sure you use a low or no-fat Caesar dressing, fat free croutons, and go easy on the salt. Along with the salad, you can eat six whole wheat crackers, an orange or an apple (or any other fruit really) and a cup of low-fat milk.

For dinner you can enjoy a broccoli stir fry. For instance, you can add a cup of broccoli, a teaspoon of sesame oil, half a cup of peppers, half a teaspoon soy sauce, three ounces of tofu and a third of a cup of walnuts. Next to this tasty dish you can serve a cup of brown rice, with a whole wheat roll and a tablespoon of honey. Enjoy it all with herbal tea.

In addition, you have room for one snack whenever you feel the need for it. For instance, you can eat two rye wafers with 1.5 ounces of cheddar cheese (low fat), and a six-ounce glass of pineapple juice.

As you can see, creating a balanced menu isn't all that hard if you follow the dietary guidelines. Let's take a look at another example.

Example 2

By following the same guidelines we established earlier, we can manage to create a 1,800 calorie menu.

For breakfast you can have an English muffin, with two tablespoons of fruit spread, and a banana. You can also drink a cup of low-fat milk.

For lunch, enjoy a burger made with three ounces of lean beef, tomatoes, lettuce, and whole wheat bun. Along with it, you can have a tossed salad with two tablespoons of a low or no-fat French dressing. To finish it off, you can also enjoy an ounce of pretzels and 16 grapes. Counting grapes may seem over the top, but you don't have to count them precisely. Just fit them in according to your calorie requirements.

As for dinner, try some lean chicken with couscous veggie salad. You can also have a whole grain roll with a tablespoon of honey, an orange, and a cup of milk.

As for the daily snack, you can opt for a banana and a cup of low fat yogurt.

What Not to Eat

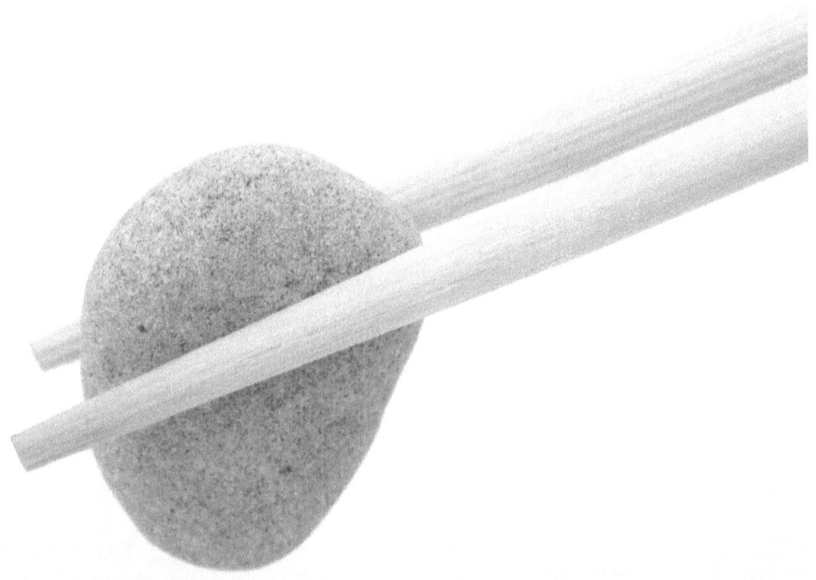

So far, we've mostly discussed what we should eat to stay healthy, fit and lose weight. While the focus of this book is to eat healthy and nutritious foods, that doesn't mean you should entirely give up on those that are considered unhealthy.

Going cold turkey isn't the solution because you might end up being haunted by multiple cravings and those are so hard to resist that you'll end up feeling frustrated and on the edge. Resistance is futile! We like to eat, food makes us happy, but we also need to stay healthy. So instead of going from one extreme to another, we need to find the right balance. If you feel the need to enjoy some potato chips or an ice cream, you can still have that. The key is portion control and frequency.

You can eat your favorite foods and snacks. However, you should account for their calories and don't eat them on a daily basis. For instance, some bodybuilders like to have a cheat day once every two weeks. Some of them even once a week. It all depends on what you're cheating on your diet with.

The first thing you need to avoid is added sugar. The key word here is "added" because not all sugars are evil (we'll talk more about this in a later chapter). If it's white sugar, brown sugar, molasses, or corn syrup, you need to eliminate it all if possible, or at least move it to the cheat list. You should consume these sugars rarely because they offer no nutritious value besides carbs. In addition, they are high calorie sources. Just grab a bottle of Coke (the original, not diet or zero) next time you go to the store and check the number of calories on the label. You'll be shocked. This is one of the reasons why so many people are overweight. They don't think to check how much a soda is worth in calories. Some people even think that drinks can't make you fat and they drink an entire two litre bottle of coke every day.

Drinks that are listed as "natural" are also in the same boat as sodas. So, try to squeeze your own orange juice instead of buying in the store. Most of it has added sugar and therefore a lot of calories.

While we're still in the sugar category, you should also avoid all the baked sweets like doughnuts, cookies, and pastries of all kinds. However, you can still enjoy them once in a while on your cheat day, especially if you make them at home. The problem with these products isn't just the added sugar. They also contain a high amount of fats and salt (even when you don't feel it because of the sugar). There are plenty of recipes online on how to bake cookies without adding any sugar, or by using sugar substitutes.

Next up we have fatty meats and all processed forms of it. You don't have to quit your grilled pork chops and ribs for good, but you should limit their consumption. Make the portions smaller, and eat these fatty products only once or twice a month. In addition, the processed meats usually contain a very high amount of sodium that's not good for you. Replace these products with skinless chicken, beans, soy, peas, lentils, nuts, and fish.

Now let's talk about that sodium. Salt is absolutely necessary for human life. It's so important for our health that the Romans used it as a form of currency sometimes. As a fun fact, the word "salary" comes from "salarium" in Latin. Its root word is "sal" which means salt. Sodium is found in nearly every product these days because it makes everything taste better. It's also a cheap commodity, so many companies use it to make their low-quality products taste better. Because of this it's quite common for people to consume around 3,500 milligrams of sodium, which isn't good. Remember that the limit's at around 2,400 milligrams.

Eating so much salt is a big problem because such large amounts of sodium on a regular basis can cause various heart diseases, strokes, and raise blood pressure in general. When purchasing various foods, especially processed ones, you should check the label and see how much sodium is found in one serving. Fortunately, if you like to eat salty foods and you're having trouble lowering the amount of sodium in your diet, you can try salt replacements. Salt is just sodium chloride and it can be replaced with salt that contains mostly potassium chloride instead. This potassium-based salt tastes almost the same as the sodium one, but it's not bad for your heart.

Summary

In this chapter you learned how to plan your meals and your diet in general. This part might seem overwhelming perhaps, but if you plan ahead, you will save yourself a great deal of time and headaches. So, go through this chapter once again in order to solidify everything you need to know. Once you have all the tools, you can easily build up your diet your own way and enjoy food without cravings and without returning to your old ways.

In addition to knowing what to eat, knowing how to shop is just as important. Stores and companies know how to advertise and lure in their customers. They gather years worth of data on their customers' spending habits, eating habits, preferences, and much more. They know you so well that sometimes you don't even realize they're trying to draw you in. So, plan your shopping as well. Don't go to the store hungry and buy what your healthy diet demands.

Chapter 5: Are Fat and Meat
Good or Bad? Yes!

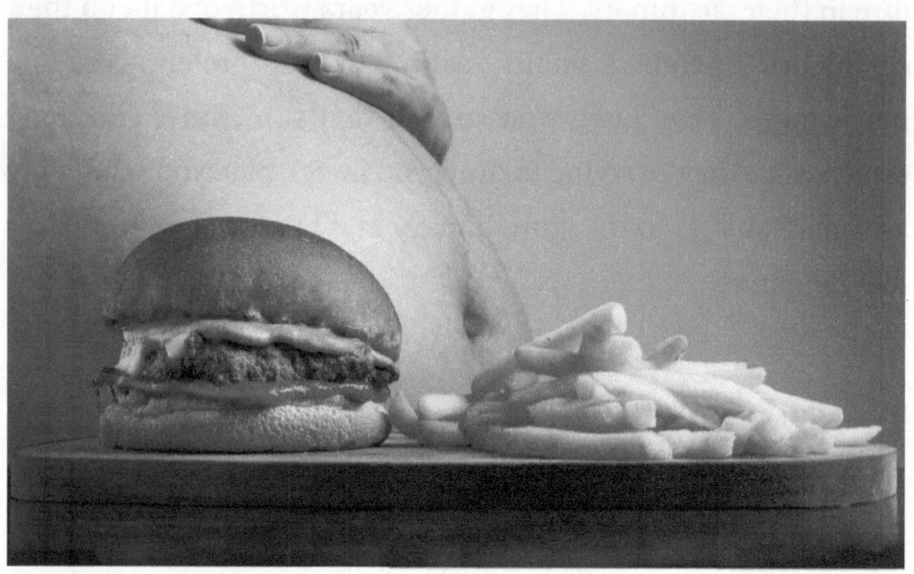

"You want to lose weight? Just don't eat fat." How often did you hear this from your friends or family? We are always told in order to lose fat we have to stop consuming it. It's an age old myth from the times when fat was just a three letters word. Since then we learned so much more. And yes, it might work when it comes to losing weight, but you won't get any healthier by eliminating it completely from your diet. In fact, you might even start to feel worse. This is because our bodies actually need fat in order to function properly.

Fat also helps us absorb some of the vitamins and minerals vital to our wellbeing. They also serve as the building blocks for the cell membranes because they act as a skin, or protective layer of the external parts of the cells. Fats also act as a "shield" (the myelin sheath) that surrounds our nerves. Without fat, our blood wouldn't clot, muscles wouldn't move and inflammation would go on a rampage through our bodies. Fats are needed in our bodies, and we need to consume them in order to stay healthy. But what does that mean for losing weight? Is it as simple as being moderate in eating fatty foods?

Well, the answer is much more complicated, although it's good advice to be moderate in anything we consume. When it comes to fat there is more than one type, and some types are good and others bad for us. In fact, there are four types of fats we have to be aware of when choosing our food. Monounsaturated and polyunsaturated fats are generally considered good for us, while trans fats are bad. There are also saturated fats which can be beneficial, but we have to be wary when consuming them. They are somewhere in the middle, between good and bad.

What makes all these fats so different? They are all made up of carbon and hydrogen atoms anyway. However strange it sounds, it's the length of the chain that these carbon and hydrogen atoms make, as well as the number of hydrogen atoms connected to one atom of carbon that makes all the difference. Even though this sounds like a really unimportant and very slight difference, it translates into a very different form and function of each type of fat.

All fats are derived from fatty acids of which some are essential for good health. By consuming certain types of fats, our bodies are able to transform them into fatty acids which will improve our wellbeing. But let's not get ahead of ourselves. Instead, let's look at all the types of the fats, one by one, summarize how and why they are good or bad for us, and see all of the benefits they bring to our bodies.

Trans Fats

These fats are also called trans-unsaturated fats, or trans fatty acids and are considered bad for us. In very small amounts they can be found in meat and milk. However, the main source of trans fats comes from vegetable oils. The discovery of trans fats was purely accidental as it's a byproduct, or a leftover of industrial processing other types of fats. Today, it's used in the snack food industry such as chips or popcorn. It's also used for frying fast food and in producing packaged baked products.

Trans fats are derivative of the process known as hydrogenation which is used to turn liquid oils into solid fats in order to preserve them and not to allow them to go rancid. Trans fats have no health benefit whatsoever, they are indeed bad for us and they are banned in some countries. As mentioned previously, the

United States effectively banned usage of trans fats in the food products and restaurant servings. Other countries chose to regulate the amount of trans fats in their food servings. In the European Union, the allowed amount is maximum 2g of trans fat per 100g of fat (European Commission, 2019)

How exactly are trans fats influencing our bodies? Why are they considered so bad that they are being banned? They are playing an important role in increasing the risks of coronary artery disease, where the blood flow to the heart is reduced because of the plaque that builds up in arteries. This disease is the most common among all heart ailments. Coronary artery disease is also one of the most common causes of death around the world.

Trans fats raise the levels of low-density lipoprotein which is known to us as "bad cholesterol." At the same time, they lower the levels of high-density lipoproteins, which we call the "good cholesterol." They also increase triglycerides in the bloodstream and play a role in promoting inflammation in our bodies which can lead to other heart diseases, stroke, diabetes and other chronic conditions.

Simply put, we do not have a need for trans fats at all and we shouldn't consume it. However, it's really difficult to avoid as they are commonly found in popular products such as margarine or shortening. The best thing you could do is limit your intake of trans fat to no more than 2 grams per day. All producers are required to note how much trans fats can be found in their products. However, one product can also contain trans fats if the label doesn't mention them. They can be hidden in writing such as "partially hydrogenated" in the ingredient list. It means the producer uses oils which went through a process to make them solid, and they contain trans fats. Trans fats can also be written as trans fatty acids, and you should be aware that it means the same thing, therefore you should avoid that as well.

Avoiding trans fats doesn't mean condemning yourself to unflavored food which will just provoke cravings in you. It all comes down to food choices you make and they can be both healthy and tasty. Avoid food that has a high caloric value but low nutritional value. These are often foods with lots of sugar, snacks, full blown meals or beverages. To name a few, avoid: cookies, pies, donuts, biscuits, crackers, packaged breads, frozen meals, ice creams, milk shakes, chips, fast food, shortening and margarine, creamers that are non-dairy and so on. If you are a vegan, beware of the products that are marketed specifically to you as vegan food as they can contain trans fats. Be careful to read labels and make the right choice.

There are better choices out there that are not using any trans fats. If you like to cook, you will always be able to find recipes which use oils instead of solid fats. Avoid using shortening, butter or margarine whenever possible and opt for sunflower or olive oil. If you love your spreads, choose softer ones as they contain much less trans fats then harder spreads. Even soft margarine today contains less than 1% of trans fats and it's a good substitute for hard margarine which is commonly used in households. Avoid consuming commercially prepared cakes, pies and pastry. Instead, bake at home and have full control of the ingredients you are using. When frying food, use low trans-fat oils like safflower or cottonseed oil. Avoid buying blended vegetable oils in supermarkets even if they are labeled as mono or polyunsaturated as they will contain trans fats due to the refining process.

Even though the main source of trans fats are industrially processed oils, they can be found in nature, too. There are trans fats in dairy products and the meat of ruminants (cows, sheep and goats) which are capable of fermenting food in their digestive system prior to digesting it; these trans fats are called vaccenic acid. However, these naturally occurring trans fats showed different characteristics than industrial ones. In fact, vaccenic acid might be beneficial as it lowers total triglycerides and bad cholesterol. Unfortunately, it also lowers good cholesterol which might be problematic.

Mammals are capable of transforming vaccenic acid into rumenic acid and as such it has the potential to combat cancer. However, more studies are needed. Not all is good when it comes to vaccenic acid, as it turns out, bipolar disorder and schizophrenia patients have elevated levels of it in their system. Because of insufficient data on animal based trans acids, it's usually advised that all trans fats should be considered equally harmful. This is why their consumption needs to be reduced to trace amounts. I encourage you to eat more poultry or fish instead of red meat, and lower the consumption of dairy products as much as you can.

Saturated Fats

Saturated fats are somewhere in between good and bad. For most people it's advised to keep the consumption of these fats to under 8% of your daily intake. This is because saturated fats can drive cholesterol up which, again, can lead to coronary artery disease.

Saturated fats are solid at room temperatures. Most animal fats are saturated. Think how bacon grease gets solid after it cools off and you will get the idea. Some saturated fats are plant based, like coconut or palm oil. The greatest sources of saturated fats are any fatty meat, chicken with skin or dark chicken meat, butter, cream, and cheese. In fact, all dairy products that are made out of whole milk contain large amounts of saturated fats. Nuts are also rich in saturated fats. If you want to lower the amount of saturated fats you consume from red meat you can substitute it with fish or skinless chicken breast. You can still consume beef, pork or lamb but choose the parts that are not greasy.

Lean meat will still contain saturated fats but in much lower quantities. If you are cooking using animal fat, think about replacing it with vegetable oils, but be cautious and do not opt for tropical oils such as palm kernel oil or cocoa butter. As with trans fats, saturated fats are commonly found in prepared foods such as pizza, snacks, deserts and meat products such as sausages and bacon. Producers are obliged to label saturated fats too, and it will be easy for you to make good choices when grocery shopping. However, they can come under different names such as lauric and myristic acids which are most commonly found in tropical oils, or as palmitic and stearic acids commonly found in cocoa, nuts, eggs or meat.

Unsaturated Fats

Healthy fats are always liquid at room temperature and they mainly come from vegetables, nuts, seeds and fish. The division between monounsaturated and polyunsaturated fats is mainly chemical, but they do have different health benefits too. While monounsaturated fats are keeping us at low risk of heart diseases, polyunsaturated fats are required for our whole bodies to work properly.

Monounsaturated Fats

Monounsaturated fats can be found in vegetable oils such as peanut, canola, olive and avocado oil. Most nut oils and high-oleic safflower or sunflower oils are rich in monounsaturated fats too. In 1960 scientists did something called the Seven Countries

Study where they compared lifestyles, diet and the number of strokes and coronary disease from patients of different regions in order to find the causes of these diseases.

Seven countries were chosen in four regions of the world: the United States, Northern Europe, Southern Europe and Japan. The study was successful in making a correlation between high cholesterol and increased risk of coronary heart disease. The findings suggested that people of the Mediterranean areas are healthiest and have significantly lower numbers of heart disease and stroke patients than others. The Mediterranean Diet is accepted as being the healthiest and it's known for higher levels of monounsaturated fats through usage of olive oil and fish. Don't forget to check out the Mediterranean pyramid again if you want to follow this diet.

However, Mediterranean people are more and more influenced by western eating habits and because of that the risk of related diseases is increasing. This, unfortunately, serves to confirm the correlation between the diet and risk of heart attack or stroke. Other diseases that are being affected by the Mediterranean diet rich in monounsaturated fats are cancer, type 2diabetes, neurodegenerative diseases and so on. However, it's not recommended to increase intake of monounsaturated fats but instead to substitute trans fats and saturated fats with the healthier option, monounsaturated fats.

There is no recommended amount of monounsaturated fats to be consumed per day, however they do need to fit in the formula that calorie intake per day needs to contain no more than 25-30% of fats. It's best to combine monounsaturated fats with polyunsaturated fats as this is the best way to achieve balance and give your body everything it needs to function; not just properly, but healthy.

Polyunsaturated Fats

Polyunsaturated fats can be found in corn oil, sunflower or safflower oil. If you are frying something, it's most likely you are using polyunsaturated fats. The ingredients which are rich with polyunsaturated fats are fish, oysters, seeds and nuts. Another name for this type of fats is *essential fats* as they are required for the normal function of our bodies. However, we are not able to produce our own polyunsaturated fats and this is why they have to be consumed through food. There are two main types of polyunsaturated fats: omega-3 fatty acids and omega-6 fatty acids and both types bring specific health benefits to us.

Once more, the Mediterranean diet proved to be a better choice as it's rich in fish which is in turn rich with omega-3 fatty acids. However, if you are a vegan or simply don't like fish, there is an option for you to naturally consume omega-3 fatty acids. Marine algae are excellent sources of these essential fats and lots of products available contain them. You can also opt for supplements made completely out of Marine algae just make sure you do your research and choose the best quality ones. Other sources of omega-3 fatty acids are: walnuts, edible seeds, algal oil, hemp oil, soybeans and so on.

The health benefits of both omega-3 and omega-6 fatty acids are numerous however, supplementing them doesn't influence the risk of all-cause mortality. There is also no correlation found between these essential fats and risk of cancer, or cancer treatment. However they do lower the risk of heart attacks and of cardiovascular diseases in general. They are good for reducing blood pressure in patients with hypertension or in people with normal blood pressure.

Omega-3 is particularly showing signs of benefits to patients with rheumatoid arthritis as it reduces the need for corticosteroids. There is some evidence that polyunsaturated fats have beneficial influence on cognitive and behavioral mental problems. They also play a key role in the construction of gray matter of our brains, they stimulate our retinas and promote neurotransmissions. A correlation between essential fats and rate of premature births has been noted, but it needs further investigation.

The Role of Fats

As discussed, we need fats in order for our bodies to work properly. This is because fats directly influence our metabolism and are part of the structure of our bodies. Some fats our bodies are not able to produce on their own, and the only source comes from food. This is why when next time someone tells you to stop eating fats altogether in order to lose weight or live healthy, tell them you know better.

Energy

Fats are our main source of energy. All food is energy and by digesting it we are storing the excess energy in the form of fatty tissue. This is our energy reserve. This is where our bodies will draw energy from when there is no ready energy source (glycogen). Stored fat, or lipids, contain fatty acids, triglycerides, phospholipids and sterols. Unlike glycogen, which our body consumes immediately to burn some energy, lipids are packed together very tightly and contain no water, thus storing great amounts of energy. This energy will later be consumed by our body to give us driving force and help us our bodies function.

Energy is measured in calories, and the more calories we consume, more fat will be stored in our body. In fact, our body is so good at storing energy that we have to be careful how much calories we are consuming. All calories that are extra are not being flushed out through our digestive system as some would believe; instead they are turned into fat tissue. In order to make room for even more stored energy, our bodies will start developing fatty tissue around our organs, inside our blood vessels and in our muscles, putting stress on them, which will ultimately result in poor health. This is why we have to be mindful when consuming fats. Though beneficial, they can also endanger our health and put us at high risk of a plethora of diseases.

Regulation and Signaling Functions

Fat helps us regulate our body's internal temperature by maintaining it constant. However, people who are skinny, without much fat on them, will often feel cold. They may also constantly feel tired and will have pressure sores on their skin due to lack of fatty acids. People with excess fat will heat up more quickly. They might feel the burst of energy when doing something, but will get tired pretty quickly. In order for fat to maintain the temperature of our bodies, we need to control it and maintain a healthy balance. Lack of fat can be just as bad as having too much.

Fat also helps the body produce hormones, which regulate our appetite, our fertility and sexual drive. Women who don't have enough fat in their bodies will stop menstruating and will have difficulties conceiving. Furthermore, essential fatty acids regulate blood clotting and regulate cholesterol, which is directly correlated to many cardiovascular diseases. Fats are needed to control the possible inflammation of joints, bloodstream and various tissues. They help our bodies sustain nerve impulse transmission and play a role in storing our memories. Lipids are not just building blocks for insulating nerves, they directly influence how electrical impulses are traveling through our brain.

Insulation and Protection

The storage of fat plays more role than just that of energy reserve. Some of our organs are protected by fatty tissue; this type of fat is called visceral, and can only be found in our abdominal cavity. It protects the liver, heart, kidneys and other vital organs as well as our whole stomach. When someone has a lot of visceral fat, they have large bellies. This is different from the jiggly fat that we have in our legs or arms, which is subcutaneous fat, stored just under the skin. Visceral fat, in proper amounts, protects organs while it's the subcutaneous fat that regulates our body temperature. It also pads our certain body parts to prevent friction when they come in contact with hard surfaces (palms and buttocks). Fat also keeps us protected from external injuries, like if we fall or get hit by something.

Transporting Nutrients

When we consume fats through digestion, they break down and start to play a role in carrying important micronutrients. These micronutrients are fat-soluble which help our body to absorb them more efficiently. Nutrients that are fat-soluble and essential to our health and body functions are: vitamins A, D, E and K. Each one of them has its own important role. Vitamin A is necessary for proper function of vital organs and also improves our vision. Vitamin D brings benefits to our immune system and is also crucial for calcium absorption and bone growth. Vitamin E assists the immune system, but it also protects our cells from damage since it acts as an antioxidant. It's also helpful for cancer prevention. Vitamin K is essential for blood clotting and bone development and it also helps with the binding of calcium.

Fats also help in improving the absorption of phytochemicals from plants, such as beta-carotene or lycopene. This is why it's recommended to eat plants along with fatty foods, as that helps our bodies absorb the good nutrients. For example, olive oil on top of a salad is an excellent way to provide transportation for micronutrients from our stomach to wherever they need to go. Grain and dairy products often lose their micronutrients due to industrial processing and to compensate for that, they are often enriched. Manufacturers will add macronutrients back to processed foods in order to keep them beneficial and to increase their vitamin content.

What about Meat?

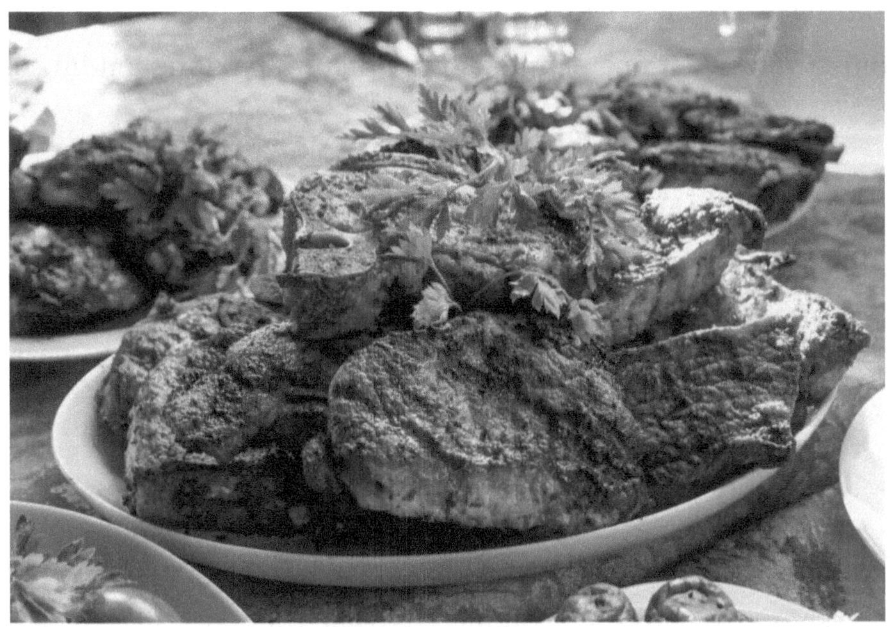

As discussed, unsaturated fats are better for us than saturated, and their main source is vegetables. But what about meat? Fat from meat consists of saturated fat. Should we all stop eating meat, even if we are not vegans? Is meat really bad for us?

To answer these questions, let's first see what role meat plays in our diet. Meat is essentially animal flesh that we cook and consume. Animal organs, called offal, that we can prepare and consume are also considered meat, but many people forget this fact. There's a reason why this is important and we will come back to it a bit later.

In the past, humans hunted for meat, but today it primarily comes from domesticated animals raised on farms. Of course, hunting is still used in some traditional societies as the main source of meat. It's categorized into different types depending on its source, and so we have:

1. Red meat - which includes beef, pork, lamb, veal, goat and game meat
2. White meat - includes chicken, turkey, duck, goose and wild birds
3. Processed meat - which consists of hot dogs, salamis, sausages, bacon, pastrami, jerky, etc.

Each meat category has its own reasons why it's good or bad for us. What they have in common is that they are all excellent sources of protein so we feel full for a much longer time and they also can speed up our metabolism. Lean meat is the most economical source of protein for humans as it contains about 25-30% protein and that's after cooking. Chicken breast, for example, contains 31 grams of protein per 100 grams, and that's after cooking. Chicken breast is considered to be one of the leanest and healthiest meats in the market.

However, if you are looking to lose weight, you should eat chicken breast without the skin, since it contains most of the calories in poultry. If you are looking to maintain your health and enjoy a healthy diet, it's good to leave a piece of skin on your chicken occasionally. It contains large amounts of unsaturated fats which can benefit your heart and general health if consumed moderately.

Protein that comes from meat is a complete protein because it contains all nine "essential" amino acids. Those are the ones we cannot produce ourselves, so we need to consume them in order for our bodies to function properly. Look at the example of 3.5 ounces (100g) of lean beef, it contains:

1. 205 calories
2. 27 grams of protein
3. 15% daily value of Riboflavin
4. 24% daily value of Niacin
5. 19% daily value of Vitamin B6
6. 158% daily value of Vitamin B12
7. 19% daily value of phosphorus
8. 68% daily value of Zinc
9. 36% daily value of Selenium

Other meats have very similar nutritional value as beef, but with much less quantities of zinc, though they can be rich in some other vitamins. For example, pork contains high values of thiamine.

Liver and other organ meats are even richer in vitamins and essential minerals, they are a great source of iron and selenium, for example. They also contain choline, a newly discovered nutrient which plays a key role in transporting fat, DNA synthesis, as well as keeping our nervous system healthy. Choline regulates heartbeat, muscle movement and liver function. Even though our bodies are able to produce our own choline, we still need to consume it in order to avoid deficiency.

Many people avoid eating organ meat because they find the thought of it disturbing. However, history teaches us that humans have consumed organs since we first started eating meat. They are still found on the menu in many societies around the world and also in some high-end restaurants, as they are considered a delicacy. Some of the poshest dishes are derived from organ meat, such as foie gras from France, made from goose liver - and sweet bread, which is nothing more than the thymus gland or the pancreas of animals. In some cultures, even animal testicles are considered a delicacy. One such dish originates in the US and has the misleading name of, "Rocky Mountain Oysters."

Organ meats are considered even more nutritious than muscle meat. They are rich in minerals, but they are also full vitamins - especially the fat-soluble vitamins: A, D, E and K. They often have fewer calories, but are richer in essential amino acids than muscle meat. They contain cholesterol, but our bodies are able to lower our own production of cholesterol if we consume enough of it. That means that by consuming it, you are not increasing your risk of heart disease. If you are having liver problems, it's best to consult your doctor as to whether or not you should eat offal meat.

Effects on Health

Recently, there has been an explosion of news warning us that red meat can cause cancer. Some studies did make a link between red meat and increased rates in colon, prostate, kidney and breast cancer. But, what the news rarely reports is that the link was made only between cancer and highly cooked meat. So, it's not the red meat that is correlated to cancer, but rather, the byproducts of high-heat preparation methods. More studies are needed to clarify the connection between cooking methods and cancer.

Processed meats have been connected to cancer, primarily of the colon. They cause inflammation which has been shown to increase the risk of cancer. For good health, it's best to avoid processed meats, they are high in salt and other preservatives. Studies that connected red meat and cancer also showed that consuming white meat does not bring us any risk. One of the studies showed that chicken breast, even cooked to the point of charring, had no connection with an increased risk of cancer.

Meat consumption has also been connected with heart disease and people are prone to blame red meat. However, there is only one study that found a weak connection between red meat and heart disease. This doesn't mean the danger isn't there. Numerous studies showed that it's processed meats that are associated with a variety of problems with heart. As for the unprocessed meat, studies show that it can either be neutral or bring benefit to the human heart. Processed meats are also connected to type 2 diabetes, as several studies showed. Nevertheless, it's the low-carb diet, which is rich in meat, that reduces blood sugar levels and is responsible for lower diabetes markers.

When it comes to consumption of meat and obesity, studies have shown there might be a connection between red and processed meat and weight gain. However, all individuals who were part of the study, consumed much more calories than it's recommended. This means that meat is not directly influencing weight gain, but it's the number of calories we consume. Many people are not aware of proper calorie calculation methods. They often include caloric value of raw meat and then they fry it adding calories with usage of oil or grease. In this case, calories from oils as well as any other sauce that might be used, or breadcrumbs, eggs and so on are not being calculated. Paleo diet shows results in weight loss even though it's rich in red meat.

Eating meat can be beneficial to our health. Consuming it makes us feel full much quicker and we need less food to satisfy our feeling of hunger. It also proved to increase metabolic rate and reduce hunger. Meat is directly linked to building up muscle mass. Although protein as such can be of any source to build up muscles, meat has other components that help the absorption of protein, stimulate growth of muscles and strengthen our joints. This is important if we are putting physical stress on our body. And it's not just muscles that are benefiting from meat. Bones are improving in density and strength when meat is consumed. One study showed that older women with a high intake of animal-based protein have a 69% decreased risk of hip fracture. Meat is also rich in iron, specifically in heme iron which is better absorbed by our body than iron from plants.

There are some tips and tricks you could follow to maximize the benefits that meat can give us, and to minimize the risks of its negative effects. It's obvious you should avoid consuming processed meats at all costs. The industrial process involves a lot of chemicals and salts which can cause kidney problems and water retention. But beside that, processed meats also have a much higher percentage of fat than a steak or a pork chop. This is because additional fat is added in order to prolong its shelf life and influence its taste.

Consider organ meats. If you are not used to the taste of these meats, try mixing them with beef, pork or chicken when cooking your regular dishes. You can also start integrating organs that have a milder taste, like heart or tongue. Balance your meals with consumption of unprocessed plant-based food alongside meat. Replace red meat with fish occasionally. Eat only lean meat even if it's ground. You can always look for the fat percentage on the packaging; try to keep it lower than 20%. Prepare lean meat in various marinades which will add to its taste and tenderize the meat. Keep in mind that marinades shouldn't contain added oils; instead try wine, soy sauce or lemon juice based marinades, with added herbs and spices. If you can't resist eating fatty meat, at least keep it for special occasions. Avoid using high-heat cooking methods when preparing your red meat, opting for slower cooking.

Summary

In this chapter you learned about fat and meat. There is a lot to explore here and that is why we had to get a bit technical. Fat is important and as mentioned before, you should never fully eliminate it from your diet. Meat is important as well, especially if it's your main source of protein. However, you should look to diversify and not make it the center of any meal. Try to switch to fish as often as possible, eat plenty of nuts, beans, and other rich protein foods. If you're a vegan, do all the above but skip the meat and fish.

Chapter 6: Fasting and Healthy Nutrition

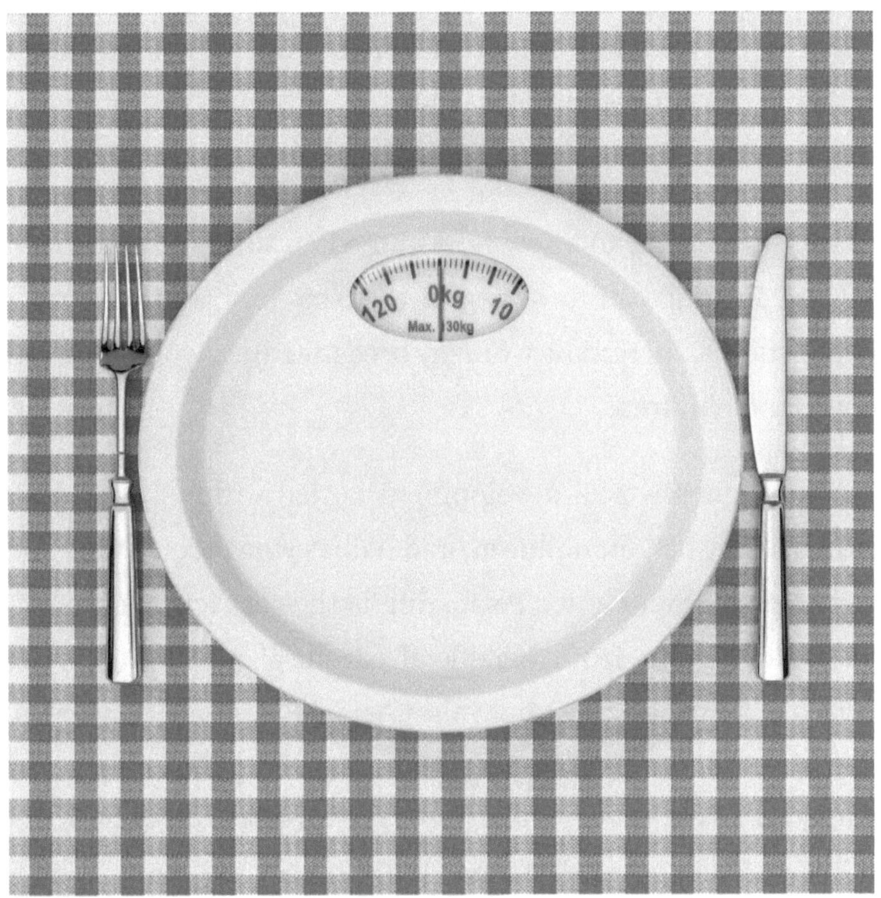

Fasting has many meanings, depending on if you are looking at it from a nutritional aspect, religious, psychological or a medical practice. What we are interested in here is the nutritional aspect of fasting, with information of how it influences our bodies from a medical aspect. In this case, fasting is the purposeful abstention from food in order to gain certain health benefits.

Fasting is more common than you'd think. Most of us have had bloodwork, and been told to fast for biomarkers like cholesterol, blood glucose and triglycerides. However, fasting also has its benefits when it comes to mental health. Some practitioners say it can improve their mood, alertness and overall feeling of wellbeing. As for weight loss, there is a special type of fasting, namely intermittent fasting; we will return to that in a little bit.

It's very important to know how and when to fast, but also who can fast. Fasting can have negative effects on certain groups of people such as pregnant women, breastfeeding women, elderly people and children.

Because their physical development is tied with what they eat, fasting is very bad for children, and babies who receive their food from their mother's milk. As fasting is the restriction of food, it means restriction from beneficial essential micro and macro nutrients. Children must not miss their daily intake of nutrients in order to develop properly. In order to stay healthy, elderly people also need to consume all of their nutrients regularly, and in a well-balanced way. When it comes to pregnant women, clearly both the mother and fetus require sufficient nutrients, so a fasting regimen is definitely not recommended.

Fasting should always be reserved for healthy people, for people who are trying to lose weight, or for people with certain medical conditions who are advised to fast by their doctors. Among people who shouldn't fast are people with a history of eating disorders, underweight people and diabetes mellitus type 1 patients. People who have a chronic disease or are taking any kind of medication should consult their doctors if they can fast.

It cannot be stressed enough that in order to start fasting properly, one must develop certain habits that will prepare the body physically and mentally for the fast. For example, sleep plays an important role in our lives. In order to maintain quality of life, we have to have enough sleep. Sleep is also important for weight loss as more sleep promotes healthy metabolism levels. However, it's the quality of food we consume which will determine if our sleep is restful, so we feel regenerated, rested and filled with energy in the morning.

For fasting, it's also recommended to get enough sun exposure as it helps our bodies to absorb certain micronutrients. Chewing food thoroughly is also important as this is the way your body will absorb more nutrients from the food. It also takes your stomach 15-20 minutes to tell your brain that you're full; so, by slowing down, you tend not to eat as much. When fasting, it's also important to maintain blood sugar levels with a high-quality diet.

There are several types of fasting which are practiced with different intentions:

1. Calorie restriction fasting: is the most basic type of fasting. This is what most people think of when they hear

the term fasting. Simply put, calorie restriction fasting is going without food for a certain period of time, usually 18-48 hours.

2. Macronutrient restriction fasting: is usually performed by athletes whose diet is quite often high in proteins. Protein puts stress on our digestive system, especially our intestines. In order to give their digestive system a break and promote healing, athletes will often put themselves on a diet of high-quality fats and carbohydrates. However, they do it only for three days, usually in periods where their activity is lowered.

3. Seasonal eating: is not really fasting but it's a type of restriction. In the past this used to be a norm for eating. You consume only what is available in the season. During the winter we would consume fattier meats and preserved food. In summer we would consume lean meat and lots of fresh veggies and fruits. Many people believe that it's the right way to do it, as certainly there should be no ripe mangoes in the northern countries during winter. The belief here is that we should eat only what season offers us, even though today's food access is much more varied.

Intermittent Fasting

Intermittent fasting is cycling between fasting and eating. It's a very popular tool for weight loss and healthy life. However, it's not a magic pill for losing those extra pounds. But, as with any other tool, if used properly, and combined with quality lifestyle changes, it will give good results. Even though it's very popular today, intermittent fasting is a very old practice, primarily via religious practice.

People today are rediscovering intermittent fasting, but often they are confusing it with starvation. Fasting is not starving yourself. Fasting is about control; you're in control of not only what you eat, but when you eat. Starvation, on the other hand, is involuntary absence of food, or in some cases pathological as in anorexia nervosa. Starving leads to many health issues, including chronic conditions and possibly death. Fasting, on the other hand, leads to health benefits and a quality lifestyle...if done right.

Intermittent fasting is best for people who have some reserves of fat in their body, as it's needed to power your body when you're not eating. Intermittent fasting will allow your body to burn the stored energy in your fat cells, and this is an excellent method for losing weight. Fasting is actually normal for the human body which is designed to work taking in account longer intervals without food. For example, normally we don't eat anything in the period between dinner and breakfast. This period is fasting, but we never give it a thought. But, the word break-fast kind of explains itself, doesn't it?

The truth is, our bodies are capable of working properly without food for longer periods of time, hours and even days. However, fasting that is longer than 48 hours is recommended only under a doctor's supervision.

But how does fasting actually work to lose weight? It's pretty simple. When we eat, our insulin levels rise in order to help our bodies store excess energy for later use. Carbohydrates are being broken down into glucose units which chain together into glycogen. This glycogen is like a battery filled with energy for later use, and it's stored in our liver or muscles. But our bodies have limited storage in which they can put these glycogen batteries. Once that storage is filled, excess glucose is now being turned into fat.

We already mentioned that fat can be stored anywhere in our body, and in reality, we have unlimited space where to store it. Fat can be stored in or around organs, muscles, blood vessels or under our skin, which is capable of constantly stretching to allow even more space. Fat is also not the best source of fuel, for the simple reason that it's used last which is why it's not easy to get rid of. Our bodies will always choose to spend stored glycogen first and only after those stores are depleted will it burn stored fat.

Glycogen can power our body anywhere between 24 and 36 hours. It's only after that period of fasting that our bodies will start using fat as an energy source. By fasting we are consciously making our bodies burn fat as we deprive it of glycogen. Today, people usually eat three meals per day leaving no time for the body to use up energy before giving it new supply. This means we are putting our body into a constant state of being fed. Our insulin level is constantly high, which won't signal our body to start burning excess energy.

Balance is achieved when we allow our bodies a proper cycle of eating and fasting. Supplying it with energy and allowing it to spend the energy stored. If this is done properly, your weight will be constant. However, if you want to lose weight, you must enter the phase of prolonged fasting to kick-start the fat burning phase. It's this amount of time we spend burning fat for energy that is called intermittent fasting.

Intermittent fasting benefits are many, including weight loss and weight control. But fasting is also sometimes called a cleansing period or detox period, because it gives the body a break, in effect. Fasting rejuvenates the body but it also clears the mind. Whether you are doing it to lose weight or to simply balance your health, you may expect some additional positive changes in your body such as: lowered insulin levels, improved concentration and mental abilities, increased energy, improved cholesterol profile, stimulated autophagy processes (cellular cleansing), a decrease in general inflammation and a boosted immunity profile.

Fasting Correctly

Intermittent fasting can be very flexible and there are different programs to serve your schedule. You can fast for short or long periods, but if you go with short stretches, you'll have to make sure you're keeping track of when you need to eat, and when you need to fast. Any long period of fasting that exceeds two days should be done only under the supervision of a doctor. Here are some predefined programs that you can choose from, or you can create your own if you feel confident enough:

1. 16:8 - This involves 16 hours of fasting and an 8 hour "eating window." This doesn't mean you should eat every hour during that time. It's about consuming your daily dose of calories during those eight hours. You can choose whether to have two or more meals, or you can even consume all calories at once. To avoid hunger, it would be best to split your calorie intake into two or three meals. For example, you can have lunch at 12:00, a snack at 15:00 and dinner at 20:00. You can also choose to have breakfast, lunch and a snack, and skip dinner if you prefer. You can organize your meals however you want as long as you do not eat anything for 16 hours after your last meal.

2. 20:4 - This involves 20 hours of fasting and a short window for eating of only 4 hours. For instance, you can eat between 3 PM and 7 PM and fast for the rest of the

day. You can either have one meal, or two smaller meals, but you have to make sure you consume enough calories so that you can carry out your normal daily activities; you don't want to pass out at work. This type of fasting is very demanding, both physically and psychologically, and this is why it's nicknamed "the warrior diet."

Both 16:8 and 20:4 are considered to be short fasts as they fit into a 24 hour day and are done every day, in order to give the best results. There are long-term fasts that last longer than 24 hours, and are done on occasion.

1. The 24-hour fast involves fasting for an entire day and having just one meal. It means you can have dinner and then again dinner the next day. Or you can choose to fast from lunch to lunch. In between you won't eat anything. You still eat daily, but only once a day. This type of fasting is recommended to be done just 2 or 3 times per week, because it's very demanding.

2. 5:2 is the most popular type of long-term intermittent fasting. It involves 5 days of eating, and 2 days of fasting. It sounds fairly easy, especially because the psychological effect is lessened this way. Anyone can be stoic enough to fast for 2 days per week, don't you think? However, there is a trick to it. Within those 5 days of eating you can eat every day but only up to 500 calories. This means your daily intake of calories is drastically reduced. You are free to choose when to eat. You can have even three meals per

day if you split 500 calories that way. You are also allowed to eat all 500 calories in a single meal.

3. Another option is alternate fasting. This is basically 5:2 with a different approach. Instead of eating for 5 days and fasting for 2, you can fast every other day. The 500 calories limit stays and you can plan your meals however you desire.

4. Next we have the 36-hour fast, which obviously means fasting for 36 hours. If you have dinner on day one, it means your next meal will be breakfast on day 3.

5. Finally, there are even more extended fasting protocols; these are fasts that last for more than 48 hours and need medical supervision. It's not recommended for weight loss unless it's prescribed by a doctor. All extended fasting places you at some level of risk. It can cause various dietary imbalances that may be fatal and this is why medical control is needed. Doctors would then check the phosphorus levels in your blood because that would indicate whether you're in trouble or not. Such imbalances occur normally in malnourished people, but there are other at risk groups such as oncology patients, elderly people, people with low energy, and of course people who are on a prolonged fasting diet.

Nutrients

People who start with intermittent fasting often make the common mistake of not eating right. They keep their old habits and hope they will lose weight as long as they spend some amount of time fasting. They often continue eating junk food during the "eating window" such as fast food or snacks that do not provide our bodies with enough nutrients, even though they are packed with calories. Not all calories are created equal, as we've covered; some foods simply don't contain all essential amino acids, vitamins and minerals we need to keep functioning properly. If you're fasting, please avoid processed foods, sweets, sugary juices, simple carbs, and sodas.

If we do not supply our body with all the nutrients it needs, it will constantly feel hungry and fasting will become a horrible experience. Satisfy your body's needs and fasting can even cause pleasure. Fasting doesn't have any different demands other than a normal healthy diet. You do not have to go far and beyond to think of what next exotic thing you should put on your plate. You need to eat a wide variety of foods in order to balance your diet and give your body all the macro and micronutrients it craves. Although there are some tricks you could resort to if you think the hunger is unbearable. Some food is simply better at making you feel full for longer periods of time, and it can still be healthy.

Eat veggies and fruits during your fast. They are rich in fiber and can fill you up. Beans and legumes are also amazing at keeping the hunger away and they are rich in protein. Include black beans and chickpeas during your fast and you will notice how easy it's to stay full. Be careful with nuts though. They are filled with antioxidants and unsaturated fats, but they are also very high in calories and can easily make up most of your daily needs. Be modest with nuts in order to give your body what it needs, but also to keep the calorie count low.

If you are a meat eater choose lean beef, white meat and seafood. They are all amazing sources of protein. Be sure to prepare them in the right way so you don't add calories which don't really benefit you nutritionally. Avoid deep frying, for example, and if you like roasting your meat, keep it above the tray so that the fat can melt away. This method is really helpful when roasting a chicken with skin, as there will be no excess fat.

In addition, you can eat eggs as they are also a good source of protein. Seafood is rich in omega-3 and 6 amino acids which are very beneficial for our health. Add salmon, shrimps and trout to your weekly menu and you will fend off heart disease, depression and risk of dementia. Include whole grains as well, during your fast. They are also rich with protein that keeps us satisfied, but they are also rich with fiber. Choose whole grain bread and brown rice. Try out some new grains, such as ancient grains like sorghum, spelt or kamut. You might like them more than other whole grain products and find a way to incorporate them in your diet on a regular basis. Remember that low-fat dairy products have a lower nutrient profile, so you might want to avoid them, or eat smaller serving sizes of dairy products. You don't have to give up cheese or yogurt, just be careful with how many calories you consume and it will be fine.

Drinking and staying hydrated is essential for fasting. You should drink plenty of water to keep yourself hydrated throughout the entire day. Water has no calories so drink as much as you can. However, water isn't the only drink you are allowed to have. Feel free to have zero-sugar beverages, be it tea or coffee but make sure not to use any cream or sugar.

If you opt for zero sugar sodas, be aware they contain artificial sweeteners which may trigger your sugar cravings. This doesn't mean it will happen, but best to stay away from them if you struggle with fasting on a psychological level. I highly recommend you avoid them altogether, as they also trigger an insulin response in your body, which increases inflammation and can actually cause you to store fat.

Another good source of liquid and nutrients that you might want to implement in your diet is bone broth. This is a great option for your fasting periods and it will help you fight off the feeling of hunger. Not only that, it's packed with great vitamins and minerals, it can really help you stay healthy during fasts, and just in general. It's super easy to make - take the bones of any meat product, like chicken, turkey, beef or pork, add some root vegetables like potatoes and carrots, along with other veggies (maybe celery, spinach, etc.). Simmer it all together, in enough water to cover everything (don't forget to add some salt and pepper) for several hours. When done, strain the bones and vegetables off, retaining the liquid in a pot. Transfer the broth to a storage container, and you have your bone broth.

And last, but not least, it's important to create a productive and practical routine around your fasting program, whichever you choose. Practicing discipline will help you with intermittent fasting as you will easily fight off any cravings, the feeling of hunger and possible "blue days" when you feel under the weather. You should train your body to know when to expect food and when not to, so it will know when to send you the signals of hunger. Of course, it takes time to create this habit and you must be persistent and consistent. Eat as healthy as possible to help your body get used to the new diet and poised to start burning off excess fat. If you follow this simple guideline you can expect not just to lose weight, but to also feel healthier and more energetic.

Summary

In this chapter we focused on fasting. Many people already fast because of religious reasons or because they read somewhere that it's a good way to lose weight. However, fasting can be dangerous if done incorrectly. That is why it's recommended for you to consult a doctor or a dietary specialist before going on a fasting period, especially if it's an extensive one. Use the information in this chapter as a guideline if you're a healthy adult, but are aware of some problems, consult a specialist to make sure intermittent fasting is a worthwhile option for you to pursue.

Chapter 7: Snacks Can Be Nutritious

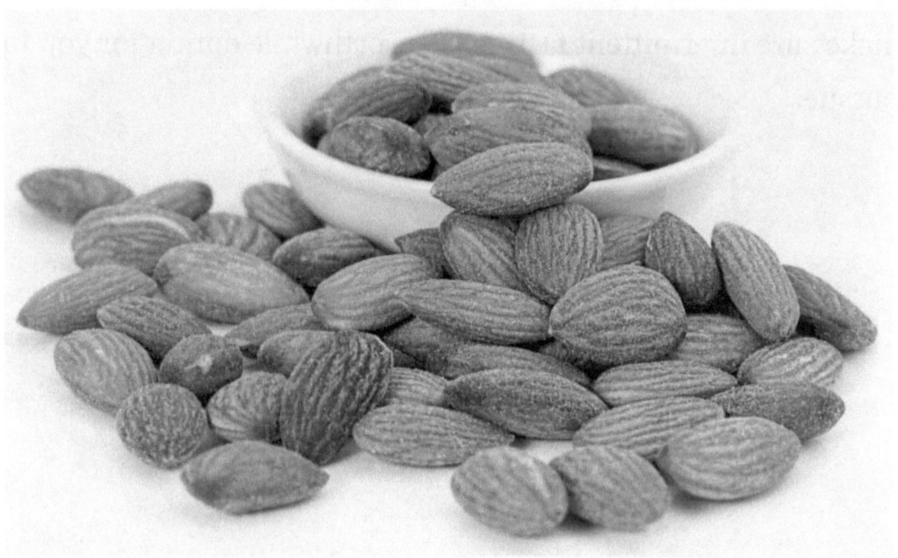

Snacking is something you should avoid if you're trying to lose weight. However, it can be beneficial if our calorie counter has room for a small snack or two. Healthy snacks can offer the vitamins and minerals we are missing. If prepared in the right way, they can also be low in calories and not influence our daily recommended levels of calories by much.

People are used to snacking in between meals. Unfortunately, they go for industrially processed, prepackaged foods with little to no nutritional value. If you want to work on new habits and change your lifestyle to a healthier one, forget about chips, popcorn, processed sweets, and sugary sodas. Think healthy in order to benefit from your snacks. What is first to come to your mind? Fruit, vegetables and nuts make awesome snacks. They are rich in vitamins, fiber and antioxidants (though you have to be careful with nuts as they are high in calories). If prepared properly, healthy snacks are good for any occasion, such as school, office, and movie night, or even a party. Healthy doesn't have to be boring.

When it comes to healthy snacks, you should avoid buying them from the supermarket. Some companies do make healthy snacks, but it's best to avoid them as they can contain artificial sweeteners or extra salt to help with the preservation. Best option is to plan your snacks in advance and make them yourself. If you make them well in advance and store them properly in your fridge or sealed containers, they will be ready to grab whenever you feel like snacking and need an extra boost. Prepare the ingredients in advance and shop in bulk in order to have everything ready when you're in the mood to spend some time in the kitchen. Keep them fresh by using vacuum sealed containers and zip bags. They are excellent at keeping your snacks from getting spoiled quickly and are easy to carry whenever you're in a rush.

There is this term nutritionists like to use for people who are constantly snacking and it's kind of funny. The term is "grazing" as it reminds us of livestock or wild animals that are constantly munching on grass. But these animals have different diets and that is what's natural for them to stay healthy. It's not for humans. You have to keep away from constantly snacking.

People who "graze" often don't even pay any mind to what they are eating and they lack essential nutrients. It's precisely this lack of nutrients that keeps them in a vicious circle and constantly in the need to munch on something.

If, instead, they would pay attention to consuming the right healthy foods, they would stop feeling this way. Grazing not only adds calories which will end turn into fat, but it expands the stomach. The larger the stomach, the more hungry we feel. If you're a person who often "grazes," stop immediately. Ask yourself what is good for you and what might your body miss. Opt for a healthier snack, like a fruit, a veggie or handful of nuts, for instance. You will be surprised how much better your body will feel.

Another mistake people often commit when snacks are involved is the serving size. Even when they are as healthy as they get, too much of them can do more harm than good. Just like with proper meals, snacks have calories and if you eat too much you will gain weight. It's recommended to consume one quarter of our daily calories from snacks, if possible, less. Serve snacks in small bowls or tea plates so you have a better control of the quantity you eat. Eat them slowly as it will help you feel full. If you allow some time between the bites to pass, the signal that says, "hey, I have food in me" from your stomach will pass to your brain and in return the brain will signal your stomach saying "ok, that's enough." Try it out, eat slower and see how full you feel by the time your plate is almost empty.

Snacks don't just serve as gap fillers between the meals and they don't provide us only with extra nutrients. They also provide comfort and play a significant role in our mental health and how we feel.

Snacks can be comfort food even when they are healthy. We tend to eat more in moments of sadness or anxiety. Food brings comfort and we shouldn't deprive ourselves from it. But we need to pay close attention to what we eat and in what amounts. Snacks also potentially provide us with higher concentration of nutrients, thus providing more energy than a typical meal might. They are often tools for people with special physical needs. For example, certain snacks are helpful when you need to concentrate (higher in protein), while others are great for keeping energy levels when exercising or recovering from physical work activities.

Here are some healthy recipes for snacks you can prepare at home on your own. There are a ton of resources online, too. For example, many celebrities are aware of the benefits of snacking and they can serve as an awesome source for recipes. Just look at their figure! They certainly don't stay in great shape by binge eating processed junk food. There are also great internet bloggers and influencers who have a lot of great information on healthy snacks and meals - but, make sure you are following the guidelines of the food pyramid you chose to adhere to.

Aside from listening to others, once you get some experience you can start experimenting and creating your own recipes. Keep a book of the recipes you liked and prepare them as often as you can. Don't forget that snacks should come in a great variety as well.

Beetroot Chips

For this recipe you will need:

1. 2 beetroots, washed and peeled
2. 3 tablespoons of olive oil
3. 2 teaspoons of kosher salt
4. Black pepper as much as you like it
5. Roughly chopped rosemary, amount according to your taste
6. 1 teaspoon of cumin

Preparation method:

Prepare two trays with baking paper while preheating the oven to 200°C. Cut the beetroot as thin as you possibly can. You can do it manually with a knife, or you can use a handheld slicer. Use a mixing bowl to mix your slices of beetroot with all the spices and olive oil. Mix well to make sure every slice is coated with the mixture. Place each separate slice of beetroot on the baking paper and make sure they don't touch each other. The thinner the slice, the less time it will need to bake. Check on them often so they don't burn.

Bake them approximately 15 minutes, until you see they become crispy. If you store them in an airtight container, they can last for several days out of the fridge. Using the same method and even the same spices you can make apple chips or sweet potato chips by following similar steps. For the sweet version you can sprinkle the apple slices with cinnamon and a little bit of sugar instead, and you don't even need to add oil.

Banana Ice-Cream

This is a one ingredient recipe that will have the same texture as ice cream, but without any milk and added sugar. You can use as many bananas as you want. Slice them up and freeze the slices, spread on baking paper. Just make sure there's room in between the slices so they don't stick. This is done so the bananas easily fit in the blender later. Once your bananas are frozen, blend them in a food processor until they are creamy. The ice cream is ready to eat immediately while the rest you can divide in portions and freeze for later use. Just allow the portion to start melting before eating.

Low Calorie Blueberry Muffins

For this recipe you will need:

1. 1 cup all-purpose flour
2. 1 tablespoon all-purpose flour (keep separate from the previously prepared cup)
3. 1 cup rolled oats
4. 2 teaspoons of baking powder
5. A pinch of salt
6. 2 eggs, beaten lightly
7. 1 cup Greek yogurt
8. 1/3 cup of honey
9. ¼ cup of low-fat milk
10. 2 teaspoons of vanilla extract
11. 1 cup of blueberries (frozen or fresh)

Preparation method:

Use silicone liners for the muffin tray. This way you won't have to grease the tray and add extra calories. Start by mixing 1 cup of flour with oats, baking powder and salt in a large mixing bowl. In another bowl mix the whisked eggs, yogurt, honey, milk and vanilla extract. Now you can add the liquid mixture to the dry one and stir it to create a batter. Wash the blueberries if they are fresh and roll them in the remaining tablespoon of flour. This will keep their moisture in, so the batter can bake properly. Fill your muffin tray with batter to the top. Bake in a preheated oven at 350F for 15-20 minutes. Use a toothpick or a fork to check whether the muffins are done. If the toothpick comes out of the muffin clean, your sweet snack is ready.

Tuna-

Stuffed Celery Sticks

This is an awesome party snack, or for lazy football Sundays, when you spend time with your family and friends.

For this recipe you will need:

1. 1 can of tuna fish packed in water
2. 1 tablespoon of Greek yogurt
3. 1 tablespoon of sauce for wings (any brand you prefer)
4. 3 celery sticks
5. Black pepper according to your taste

Preparation method:

Mix the tuna in a bowl together with Greek yogurt, wing sauce and black pepper until a smooth pate like texture is achieved. Wash and cut the celery sticks to the preferred size and fill them with the tuna filling. It's that easy to prepare a healthy snack! You can store the mixture in an air-tight container in the fridge if you prepare larger quantities for later, but do not keep already filled celery sticks. Better to use them fresh each time you crave them.

Chickpeas on Toast

This is the healthy version of the very popular British snack simply known as beans on toast. This snack is faster to make as it requires no cooking time.

For this recipe you will need:

1. 1 slice of whole-wheat or sprouted wheat toast
2. ¼ cup of canned chickpeas
3. grated carrot, according to your taste - add as much as you think you'll need
4. 1 teaspoon of olive or sesame oil if you want to add flavor
5. 1 tablespoon of freshly squeezed lemon juice
6. Salt and pepper according to your taste

Preparation method:

Mash the chickpeas and mix with sesame or olive oil using a potato masher. You can also use a fork or whisk as the mass needs to stay chunky but spreadable. Add lemon juice, salt and pepper and mix well. Add grated carrots to the mix and done! Just spread it on your toast. You can decorate this snack with some parsley if you like. The topping can be kept in an air-tight container in the fridge for later use. Avoid storing already spread toast as it will get mushy and your yummy snack will be ruined.

Summary

In this chapter we discussed how snacks can be quite useful to a healthy diet. They might not be the best if you're trying to lose weight, but even then, you can get away with a healthy snack if you use the right recipe, and are following the calorie counts. I hope you enjoy exploring the handful of recipes included, try them out and modify them as you wish. Don't forget to look online for other great recipes. A simple search for "Keto Friendly Snacks," for example, will bring up a ton of options.

Enjoy!

Chapter 8: What about Sweets?

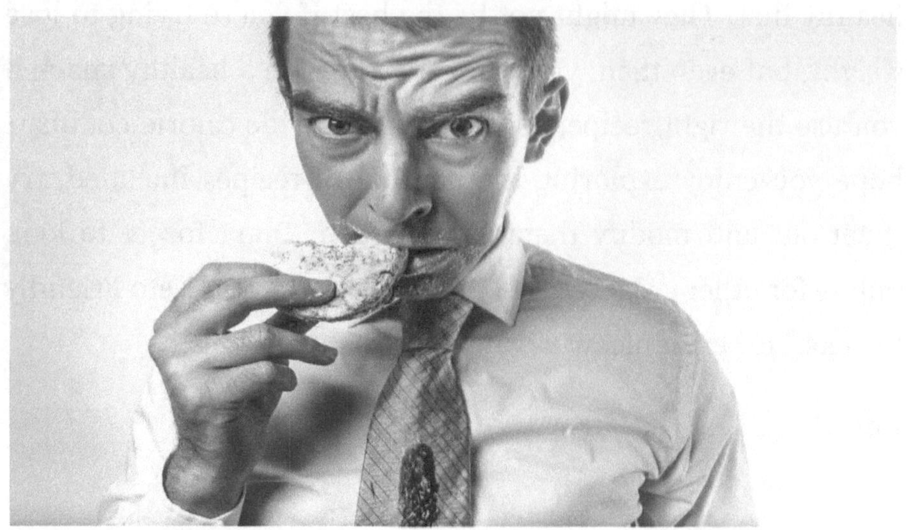

We're all repeatedly told that sweets aren't healthy and we shouldn't eat them, especially if we're trying to lose weight. And I am sorry, but this is all true. The healthiest way to eat sweets is not to have them at all. Sweets contain tremendous amounts of sugar which is linked to type 2 diabetes and heart diseases. Sugar is one of the biggest problems when it comes to obesity in America as it's added to almost everything. Even bread contains sugar, together with all the processed sauces and marinades too.

However, it's not only sugar that's bad about sweets. Lots of them contain saturated fats which can be harmful if consumed too often, and lots of empty calories as well. This means we will consume calories that carry no micro and macronutrients that our bodies need to function properly. Now the question is, why is sugar so bad for us? Even fruit has sugar and we still recommend it when we talk about a healthy diet. So, what is the difference?

The Difference Between Fruit Sugar and Candy Sugar

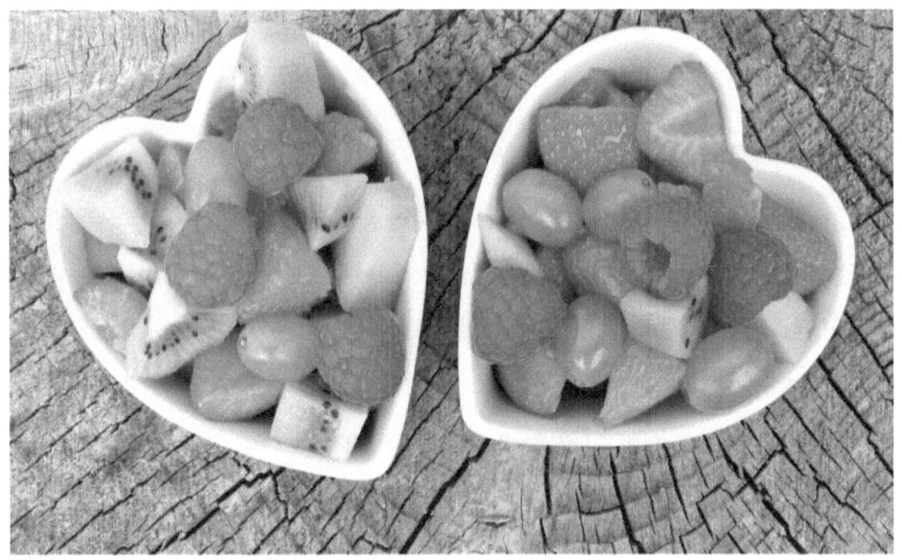

There are different kinds of sugar and it comes in many different forms when consumed through food and drinks. Sugar molecules come in two classifications: monosaccharides (glucose and fructose) and disaccharides (sucrose and lactose). We are not going to indulge in overcomplicated chemistry and explain all the types of sugars, but we are going to concentrate on what the difference is between eating a fruit and an industrially processed snack. They both contain sugar, and many people wrongly believe that fruit only contains healthy fructose, while sweets only contain unhealthy glucose or sucrose.

Fruits actually contain various types of sugar, with fructose being present in the largest quantity. Fruit also contains sucrose and glucose, so don't be fooled when someone says that an apple is pure fructose. After all, there are no good or bad types of sugar in reality. Everything bad from sugar comes from the quantities we consume. It's all in the servings! And this is exactly where the main difference between fruit and cake comes from.

Sugar is bad because we eat it in large amounts. Fruit doesn't contain so much sugar, so one serving can't have a bad effect on us. But a candy does. This is because fruit contains other nutrients which are beneficial to our bodies such as fibers, vitamins and minerals. Candy on the other hand contains large amounts of sugar while the rest are just empty calories that contain little to no nutrients. Even if presented as a "healthy" candy bar, as it might contain whole grain wheat or added vitamins, it will be so packed with sugar that it's not worth eating. I see this with some "protein" bars that have 9 grams of protein (that's great), but 30 grams of sugars (bad)!

Fructose is as harmful as glucose or sucrose. It all comes down to the amount of sugar available in fruit. Physically, it's impossible to eat an amount of fruit that will be harmful for us. What industrial candy contains is called "free sugar." This type of sugar was extracted from its natural source (fruit, cane, vegetable, grain). Extracted sugar goes through additional processing to make it attractive for consumers.

This type of processed sugar has no nutritional value to our bodies. It's easy to consume in large amounts and can lead to various health problems. One or two whole fruits are capable of satisfying our hunger, but one candy bar can't. One or two whole fruits contain a lot less sugar than a candy bar. This is the main reason why people are getting excess weight from sugar. We can't stop eating it. It's literally addictive.

Aside from not really satisfying our hunger, sugar also may cause an addiction to our brains which makes us crave even more sugar. One of the main fuels for our brains is sugar, and this is possibly one of the reasons why we can't get enough of it. The more of it we eat, the more we crave. Again, fruit does not contain enough sugar for our bodies to develop this addiction. This is why eating fruit's so much healthier than eating candy.

The recommended intake of sugar is around 50g per day. This is the equivalent to one can of soda. Even freshly squeezed orange juice is worse than eating a whole fruit. This is because for one glass of orange juice you would need to eat 4-6 whole oranges. That is a lot, and you probably can't normally eat that in one sitting. But you can drink a glass of juice in one sitting and it will contain the same amount of sugar as 6 whole oranges - but, without the fiber, vitamins and minerals.

Chances are that the food you eat while having a glass of juice is also filled with sugar. Sugar is good for the preservation of food and this is one of the main reasons why producers put it in their products. Sugar also makes food taste better. The better the taste, the more likely you are to buy the product again and again. This is why companies like sugar and put it in everything. Plus, it doesn't hurt their bottom line since sugar is a relatively cheap ingredient. This preponderance of sugar in everything might have something to do with the addictive properties of it, but that's a controversy already so we won't go there.

The conclusion is that if you stick to the recommended daily dose of sugar, you can consume it in any form. If you are in control of your sweet cravings you probably don't need to follow the advice about eliminating all sweets from your life. Just know when to stop and how to consume sugar in its most healthy form. Sugar has its own benefits if consumed right. But let's take a look at all the negative sides of sugar first.

Health Risks

Besides uncontrolled weight gain, sugar can affect our bodies in some other negative ways. The most common example is tooth decay. People often overlook this health problem because others sound so much more serious. But tooth decay is the most common disease caused by sugar. Many people argue that tooth decay is purely a cosmetic thing, but it can lead to other tooth and gum related problems that can be serious and even life threatening. After consuming sugar, it remains on our teeth and serves as food for various bacteria that live in the mouth. Bacteria love sugar so much that other food that gets stuck in our teeth doesn't even come close to causing tooth decay. When bacteria feed on sugar it produces acid that dissolves and damages our teeth. This is why it's so important to brush your teeth and remove all excess food, especially sugar, after each meal.

Because bacteria and yeast love sugar so much, our immune system might also be suffering because of it. The bacteria multiply in our bodies because we regularly supply them with sugar. Our immune system recognizes the increased number of bacteria and is trying to fight them, but it can get overwhelmed. If not functioning properly our immune system won't be able to fight off various diseases and the excess bacteria will cause various ailments throughout our bodies. It's important not to overindulge in sweets and sugary drinks when we are fighting an infection, but it's probably the best to stay away from them anyway.

Sugar also causes glucose levels in blood to spike and then to plummet. This usually leads to a false feeling of hunger. This is what we experience as a craving. When we satisfy our cravings, we don't do any service to our bodies as another glucose spike will lead to another plummet and the cycle will continue repeating. We must be strong enough and resist such urges and avoid eating sugar too often. This instability in glucose levels often leads to mood swings, headaches and fatigue. To combat them we must break the vicious cycle.

The most serious and life-threatening conditions influenced and caused by sugar are diabetes and various forms of heart disease. Sugar does not cause both types of diabetes. This is a common misconception. Diabetes type 1 is an autoimmune disease while type 2 diabetes develops from an unhealthy lifestyle. Other risk factors include genetics, sex, and age. Obesity is the number one risk factor of developing diabetes type 2 and excess sugar does lead to obesity. Once a person has diabetes of any type, eating sugar will make the symptoms of this disease worse. Insulin won't be able to regulate the levels of glucose in their blood, and if diabetes is not treated it's life-threatening. It's similar with heart disease, but sugar doesn't influence that condition quite as directly. However, added sugar contributes to obesity, high blood pressure, fatty liver disease, and other inflammatory conditions. All of these can lead to heart attacks or strokes.

As you can see, the risks that come with the consumption of sugar are many and serious. But sugar also comes with some benefits. However, it's solely on us as individuals to make a conscious decision on how to consume it, in what quantities and from which source. Choose healthy sources of sugar such as fruits and vegetables, like we talked about earlier. They have just the right amount of sugar, so we feel the benefit of that extra energy, but they are also packed with other nutrients which our bodies need. They will efficiently fight off the feeling of hunger while the processed, free sugars won't. Instead, they will drag us in a vicious circle of addiction and force us to consume it more and more.

Sugar Substitutes

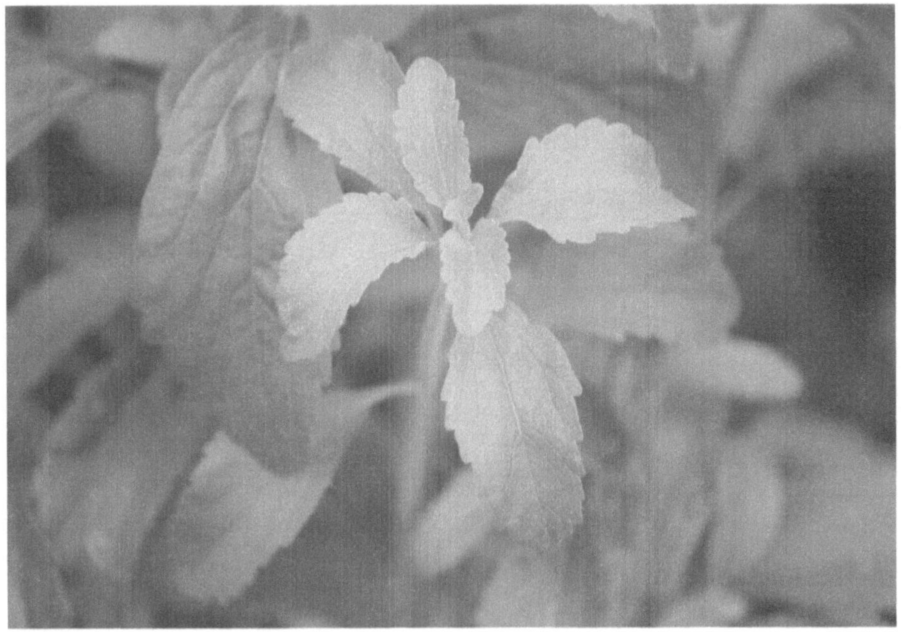

The increase of obesity and type 2 diabetes cases around the world led scientists on a quest to find the perfect substitute for sugar. The search is still ongoing even though we have a few alternatives. The perfection we are looking for would include the same taste, no calories, benefits to overall health and lack of cravings.

There are two types of sugar substitutes that exist today: sugar alcohols and high-intensity sweeteners. Sugar alcohols are sorbitol, lactitol, and mannitol. They have a similar taste to sugar and can be sweeter; anywhere between 25-100% more potent. They are often used for toothpaste and chewing gums and in lower quantities in sugar-free food. Generally, they are used in products which demand a lower quantity of sugar. This is because being alcohol-based sweeteners, they do contain calories. Most of them have 1.5 up to 2 calories per gram while sugar has 4. It's an improvement, but not enough.

If used in greater amounts, the effects of these "empty calories" will remain the same. Sugar alcohols need to be used in very low quantities if one has diabetes as it will still increase our glucose levels. Sugar alcohols are harder to digest than regular sugars. They can cause some uncomfortable side effects if consumed in excess. Because they are harder to digest, they can cause stomach aches, cramps, gas and diarrhea. Products made with sugar alcohols also contain more fat and salt which are added to replace the missing sugar.

Artificial sweeteners such as saccharin, aspartame, acesulfame, stevia or SGFE are zero or low sugar substitutes. They come from different sources and can be anywhere from 100 to 20,000 times sweeter than regular sugar. Some are natural as they are derived from plants (SGFE and stevia) and others are synthesized in labs. They are almost the perfect substitute for sugar as they are of similar taste (although some leave a metallic aftertaste), they have no calories and carbohydrates, but they may increase our cravings and some are even linked to cancer. If they are labeled as natural, that doesn't necessarily mean they are safer for consumption. Some of them can lead to digestion problems and bloating. Saccharin and aspartame are linked to cancer in some studies, but they aren't conclusive and they're discussing massive quantities of these substitutes.

Because high-intensity sweeteners have no calories, many people are quick to search for a new source of calories and thus they may even cause weight gain. If you are trying to lose weight, it's important to consume zero calories sweeteners without adding calories through other foods. If used properly, artificial sweeteners can be beneficial and promote weight loss. But, use them very sparingly - no more than one or two servings each day,

Healthy Desserts

Avoiding sugars completely is difficult and psychiatrists don't even recommend it. Sugar is needed in small amounts for a happier more fulfilled life. It gives our brains a burst of energy during which we can concentrate and work more efficiently. And honestly, it will put smiles on our faces if nothing else, due to the pure dopamine dose we receive from the sweet delight a good dessert provides us with.

The trick is, as with most foods, to balance the sugar in your diet properly, to opt for healthier substitutes, to avoid processed sugar and to not overindulge in it. If you learn how to make your own desserts, even better, since you will have a full control over the ingredients that will go in your sweets. Here are some tips and tricks you could follow to make low calorie desserts and healthier overall:

1. Choose whole-wheat flour instead of refined and processed white flour which loses some of its nutrients. Whole-wheat flour will add additional fiber to your dessert and cut the calories down. Fiber is great for a healthier digestion and a smaller number of calories will keep you on track with your diet. You can use this type of flour to make anything from muffins to waffles.

2. Use fruit instead of sugar to add sweetness to your desserts. You can add fruit to a cake and greatly reduce the amount of sugar needed. Otherwise, you can use fruit juice to add some sweetness but be aware not to overdo it as fruit juices contain more sugar than whole fruit. However, they are still a better choice than refined white sugar.

3. Use zero-calorie sweeteners. The market today is filled with zero-calorie options for making desserts. Sucralose-based artificial sweeteners come in both hard and liquid forms and you can use them to substitute sugar or syrups. They will cut the calories in your dessert as you won't need to add any sugar to them.

4. Use dark chocolate. Choose a chocolate that is at least 70% cocoa for your chocolate cake or chocolate chip

cookies. The higher the percentage of cocoa in the chocolate, the lower the sugar content.

Desserts can be tasty and satisfying even if they are low on sugar and fat. There are so many recipes for healthy desserts available online or in various cookbooks that you can't miss them. The new ways of preparing your desserts will be an adventure on its own. For instance, did you know that grilling fruit such as mango or banana brings out their sweetness and aroma even more? Imagine the possibilities if you include your own imagination whenever you make a dessert. Make a fun family day out of it and teach yourself and others how to eat healthy while still giving in to your sweet tooth.

Summary

Yes, you can have desserts and sweets, within reason of course. In this chapter we explored the difference between fruit sugars and added sugars. We also discussed the most common health risks you should be aware of. Furthermore, in this modern age we have access to a few sugar substitutes that we can use to create healthy desserts. If you follow the guidelines in this chapter you will be able to treat yourself every now and then. After all, life needs to be sweet.

Chapter 9: Counting Calories

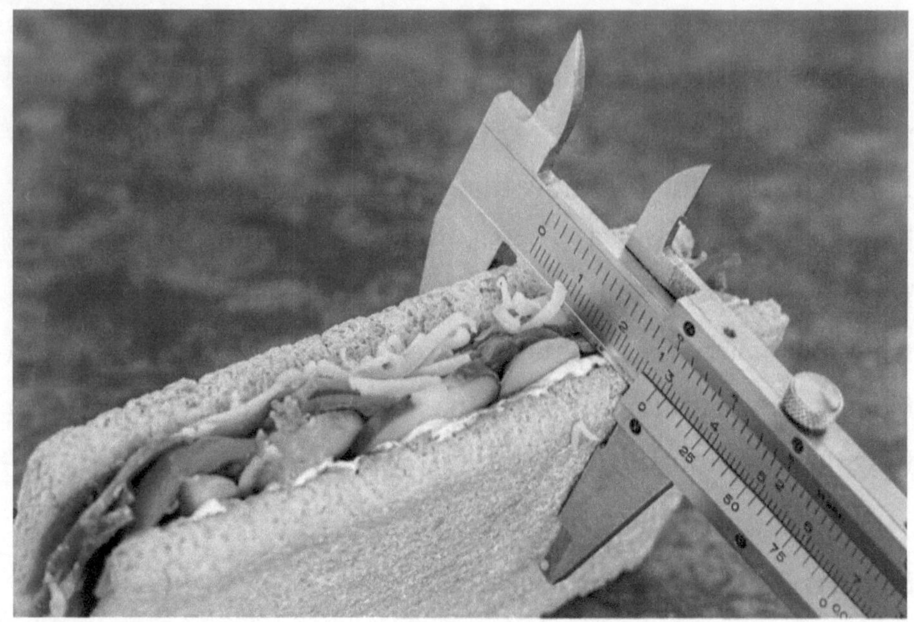

To lose weight and live a healthier life, we need to be aware of the calories we consume with each meal. But what is a calorie in the first place and why is it so important for our health?

To some extent, I am sure you already know the answer and that you are aware there is such a thing as the recommended amount of calories we need to consume over the course of a day. However, let's discuss its importance and make sure we know how to calculate the calories in the best possible way, like professionals.

Dieticians and other health experts usually talk about calories in a more casual manner. The right choice of word would be "kilocalorie" and that is what sometimes shows up on food labels in its shortened version "kcal." The kilocalorie by definition is the amount of heat needed to raise the temperature of 1 kg of water by 1 degree Celsius. We talk about kilocalories when we refer to the energy (heat) that comes from food. We aren't talking about something physical, but about a unit of measurement. We use the kcal to measure the amount of energy our bodies get from food (think of it as burning fuel for energy). Our bodies use this energy in order to perform various tasks. Even just sitting and breathing uses up energy, though in small amounts. Literally everything our bodies do, anything you can imagine requires energy that is measured in calories.

All food provides us with is calories, but not in equal ways. Healthy foods come with calories filled with nutrients that our bodies need in order to develop and function properly. They keep our organs healthy, build our bones and muscles stronger, and help us focus and memorize. Unhealthy food often comes with empty calories. This means the energy is there but without any nutrients attached to it. This is why unhealthy food often makes us feel tired and sick.

Our bodies have a limit of calories which are needed in order to satisfy our daily needs. If we consume too many calories, good or bad, the energy is converted to fat and this is how we gain weight. This is why you need to eat the right type of calories in the right amount. Of course, the amount of calories depends on the current state of your body. If you want to lose weight you need fewer calories than what your body spends in a day. This ensures your body doesn't have the fuel needed to be stored in fat. On the other hand, if you need to gain weight, simply consume more calories and if you need to maintain your weight you will eat just the right amount needed to maintain the balance.

How Many Calories?

To calculate how many calories you should eat per day, you first need to determine what your goal is. There is no magic number of calories that will guarantee weight loss or gain. We're all different and each person must calculate their own daily intake of calories. The end result depends on your current weight, sex, age, height, level of your activity and your goal.

So how does the math work? First you need to calculate your Basal Metabolic Rate (BMR). This represents the number of calories your body spends daily just for performing the basic (basal) functions such as breathing, cell production or blood circulation. To get the most accurate result you would need to do the calculations in a laboratory setting, but doing it at home won't influence your goals that much. Scientists came up with a very precise formula that will calculate your BMR easily. Here is what you need to do.

Women:

1. Measure precisely your height in inches, and weight in pounds
2. Multiply your weight by 4.35
3. Multiply your height by 4.7
4. Add the two sums
5. Multiply your age by 4.7, and then subtract that number from the sum of items 2 and 3 above.
6. Now, add 655 to what you came up with in item 5 above.

Does it sound complicated? Here is an example which will make it clearer:

Weight: 110 lbs

Height: 60 ins

Age: 20

Multiply your weight by 4.35: 110 x 4.35 = 478.5

Multiply your height by 4.7: 60 x 4.7 = 282

Add the two products: 478.5 + 282 = 760.5

Multiply your age by 4.7: 20 x 4.7 = 94

Subtract the product of your age: 760.5 - 94 = 666.5

Add 655: 666.5 + 655 = 1321.5

Your BMR in this case is 1321.5. So, if you're a woman of 20 who weighs 110 lbs and whose height is 60 inches, you need about 1320 calories just to operate your major bodily functions - this doesn't include any other activities, like walking or running.

The formula is a little different for men, but the same basic concept. Let's take a quick look.

Men:

1. Multiply your weight by 6.23.
2. Add the product of your height in inches multiplied by 12.7.
3. Subtract your age in years multiplied by 6.8 and then add 66.

Example:

Weight: 160 lbs

Height: 68 ins

Age: 25

Multiply your weight by 6.23: 160 x 6.23 = 996.8

Multiply your height by 12.7: 68 x 12.7 = 863.6

Multiply your age by 6.8: 25 x 6.8 = 170

Subtract the product of your age: 1860.4 - 170 = 1690.4

Add 66: 1690.4 + 66 = 1756.4

Now add in your activity level

If you'd like to lose weight, the next step is to determine what your activity level is. There are four types of activities and each one has its own value for the formula.

1. Sedentary people have little to no daily activity and their formula value is 1.2.
2. A light level of activity includes light exercises or sports 1-3 days per week and the value is 1.375.
3. Moderately active people who exercise or perform any sports 6-7 days per week have the value of 1.55.
4. Very active people exercise hard 2 or more times per day and the value is 1.9.

To calculate how many calories you need to consume per day in order to lose weight, you'll first need to determine how many calories you should consume to maintain your weight. You'll do this if you multiply your BMR by your activity level value.

Let's use the examples for the above. A woman who's BMR is 1321.5 and is sedentary needs to multiply the BMR value by 1.2: 1321.5 x 1.2 = 1585.8

A man who's BMR is 1756.4 and who's moderately active needs to multiply his BMR value by 1.55: 1756.4 x 1.55 = 2722.42

But this isn't all, but we're almost there!

Now you need to calculate how many calories you should subtract to lose weight. The formula is now very simple. For each pound you want to lose per week you need to subtract 500 calories. This means that if the woman from our example wants to lose one pound per week, she needs to make the following calculation:

1585.8 - 500 = 1085.8

This means she can eat 1085.8 calories per day in order to lose one pound per week.

There are plenty of online calculators that can help you determine the amount of calories needed but they are not all accurate. Pay attention to how they work and which formula they use. Some won't take in mind your age or your height but give you generic results for men and women. Others will use some other, less accurate formula and give you highly inaccurate results. The best way to calculate your own BMR and daily intake of calories is the formula above, as it was designed by scientists and is the formula that dieticians and medical professionals use.

Summary

Understanding calories is important because consuming too many will lead to obesity but consuming too little can cause other issues. That is why in this chapter you have some guidelines on how to calculate the amount of calories you need to eat depending on your goals and your personal characteristics.

Conclusion

Are you ready to embark on a new journey? You now have all the tools you need to start living healthy. You don't really need special recipes and 30-day diets and other gimmicks in order to eat healthy, live healthy and actually enjoy yourself while doing so. All you need is to understand food and how the human body works. If you take care of your body like you take care of a car, it will keep running for a long time. Do you know that old saying "we are what we eat?" It's quite accurate and if you look at people around you, you can guess pretty well what they eat just by appearance and habits.

The purpose of this guide is to arm you with knowledge. It might be tedious and even a bit scientific at times, but understanding food is important. If you get to know your body and your food, then you'll gain far more control over your lifestyle and improve it. Start living healthy today and use this book as a guide whenever you're unsure about something. With that being said, let's summarise what you've learned so far:

1. In the first chapter you were introduced to the basics of a healthy diet and optimal health. You learned that a healthy diet isn't just about the amount of calories, or the type of the diet. It's all about nutrients, variety, and balance. Remember that.

2. In the second chapter we talked about the pyramids (not the Egyptian ones). Food guide pyramids should be used as the number one guide to a healthy diet. They offer a lot of information without overwhelming you. Knowing which categories of foods to focus on and in what quantities is already a great start to a new way of life. Whether you're trying to lose weight, build muscle, or go vegan, you can use the right pyramid as a reference. Once you understand which food groups to focus on, you can start looking for the details in order to better optimize your diet.

3. The third chapter is dedicated to all the myths and misconceptions around diets, food, and weight loss, and boy are they many! We'd need an entire book just about these myths. This book only contains the most common ones, so be careful when you are ready about some "breaking news in diet!" in your Facebook feed. There's a lot of misinformation floating around and some of it's spread on purpose to profit some blog that sells the next magic pill for weight loss. Use common sense, inform yourself, and eat right.

4. In chapter four we talked about food. This is the good stuff. Learn what you should eat and how to diversify your daily menu. You can have fun eating healthy as well. Pizza and ice cream aren't the only enjoyable foods. Follow the guidelines presented in this chapter, get creative and experience food like you never have before.

5. Chapter five was when we started getting a bit more scientific. Understanding fat and meat is important, even if you're a vegan. The more you know, the better choices you can make.

6. In chapter six we explored the benefits and problems with fasting and how you can actually make it work for you. Just be careful, and if you have some kind of health issues or doubts about the whole thing, please consult a specialist.

7. In chapter seven and eight you learned about snacks and sweets. Yes, you can enjoy them on a healthy level. Nobody wants to live without experiencing some joy in eating, even when trying to lose weight.

8. Finally, in chapter eight we focused on calories. Please go over this chapter a few times since it involves a bit of math. Use the formulas to figure out how much you should eat in order to properly customize your diet.

That's it! Go forth and live healthy!

If you liked this book and you think it helped you understand healthy nutrition, please leave some feedback. If you want to read more about this topic you can also check out my other books titled "The Weightloser" and "The Keoer" found on Amazon at the following links:

https://www.amazon.com/dp/B0841N9F6Z

https://www.amazon.com/dp/B085Y7G4Q4

References

BINNS, J. (2019, December 6). Trans fat in food. Retrieved from https://ec.europa.eu/food/safety/labelling_nutrition/trans-fat-food_en

Bonaccio, M., Castelnuovo, A. D., Costanzo, S., Gialluisi, A., Persichillo, M., Cerletti, C., … Iacoviello, L. (2018, August 30). Mediterranean diet and mortality in the elderly: a prospective cohort study and a meta-analysis: British Journal of Nutrition. Retrieved from https://www.cambridge.org/core/journals/british-journal-of-nutrition/article/mediterranean-diet-and-mortality-in-the-elderly-a-prospective-cohort-study-and-a-metaanalysis/F2D6B083AA187849477112DB77820521

Bueno, N. B., de Melo, I. S. V., de Oliveira, S. L., & da Rocha Ataide, T. (2013, October). Very-low-carbohydrate ketogenic diet v. low-fat diet for long-term weight loss: a meta-analysis of randomised controlled trials. Retrieved from https://www.ncbi.nlm.nih.gov/pubmed/23651522

Capannolo, A., Viscido, A., Barkad, M. A., Valerii, G., Ciccone, F., Melideo, D., … Latella, G. (2015). Non-Celiac Gluten Sensitivity among Patients Perceiving Gluten-Related Symptoms. Retrieved from https://www.ncbi.nlm.nih.gov/pubmed/26043918

Center for Food Safety and Applied Nutrition. (n.d.). Final Determination Regarding Partially Hydrogenated Oils. Retrieved from https://www.fda.gov/food/food-additives-petitions/final-determination-regarding-partially-hydrogenated-oils-removing-trans-fat

Devries, M. C., Sithamparapillai, A., Brimble, K. S., Banfield, L., Morton, R. W., & Phillips, S. M. (2018, November 1). Changes in Kidney Function Do Not Differ between Healthy Adults Consuming Higher- Compared with Lower- or Normal-Protein Diets: A Systematic Review and Meta-Analysis. Retrieved from https://www.ncbi.nlm.nih.gov/pubmed/30383278

Evenepoel, P., Claus, D., Geypens, B., Hiele, M., Geboes, K., Rutgeerts, P., & Ghoos, Y. (1999, November). Amount and fate of egg protein escaping assimilation in the small intestine of humans. Retrieved from https://www.ncbi.nlm.nih.gov/pubmed/10564098

Harvard Health Publishing. (n.d.). The dubious practice of detox. Retrieved from https://www.health.harvard.edu/staying-healthy/the-dubious-practice-of-detox

Harvard Health Publications. (n.d.). *Counting calories.*

James, W. P. T. (1988). *Healthy nutrition: preventing nutrition-related diseases in Europe.* Cph.: World Health

Organization, Regional Office for Europe.

New study finds poor diet kills more people globally than tobacco and high blood pressure. (2019, April 25). Retrieved from http://www.healthdata.org/news-release/new-study-finds-poor-diet-kills-more-people-globally-tobacco-and-high-blood-pressure

Read "Dietary Reference Intakes for Energy, Carbohydrate, Fiber, Fat, Fatty Acids, Cholesterol, Protein, and Amino Acids" at NAP.edu. (n.d.). Retrieved from https://www.nap.edu/read/10490/chapter/10#423

Schwingshackl, L., Chaimani, A., Hoffmann, G., Schwedhelm, C., & Boeing, H. (2018, February). A network meta-analysis on the comparative efficacy of different dietary approaches on glycaemic control in patients with type 2 diabetes mellitus. Retrieved from https://www.ncbi.nlm.nih.gov/pubmed/29302846

Shams-White, M. M., Chung, M., Du, M., Fu, Z., Insogna, K. L., Karlsen, M. C., ... Weaver, C. M. (2017, June). Dietary protein and bone health: a systematic review and meta-analysis from the National Osteoporosis Foundation. Retrieved from https://www.ncbi.nlm.nih.gov/pubmed/28404575

Smith-Spangler, C., Brandeau, M. L., Hunter, G. E., Bavinger, J. C., Pearson, M., Eschbach, P. J., ... Bravata, D. M. (2012, September 4). Are organic foods safer or healthier than

conventional alternatives?: a systematic review. Retrieved from
https://www.ncbi.nlm.nih.gov/pubmed/22944875

Spector, T. D. (2015). *The diet myth: the real science behind
what we eat*. London: Weidenfeld & Nicolson.

Sutton, A. L. (2008). *Stroke sourcebook: basic consumer
health information about stroke, including ischemic,
hemorrhagic, and mini strokes, as well as risk factors,
prevention guidelines, diagnostic tests, medications and
surgical treatments, and complications of stroke ...* Detroit,
MI: Omnigraphics.

U.S. Dept. of Agriculture, Center for Nutrition Policy and
Promotion. (1996). *The food guide pyramid*. Washington, DC.

Visser, F. R. (1982). *Food composition*. Wellington, N.Z.:
Science Information Division, DSIR.

Watson, S. (2008). *Trans fats*. New York: Rosen Central.

World Health Organization. (1998). *Healthy nutrition: an
essential element of a health-promoting school*. Geneva.